This book is due for return on or before the last date shown below.

CITY OF GLASGOW COLLEGE
North Hanover Street Library
60 North Hanover Street
Glasgow G1 2BP
0141 566 4132

Homemade
BATH BOMBS, SALTS & SCRUBS
300 Natural Recipes for Luxurious Soaks

Kate Bello

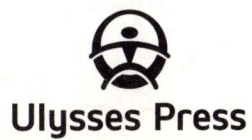

Text copyright © 2015 Kate Bello. Design and concept copyright © 2015 Ulysses Press and its licensors. All rights reserved. Any unauthorized duplication in whole or in part or dissemination of this edition by any means (including but not limited to photocopying, electronic devices, digital versions, and the Internet) will be prosecuted to the fullest extent of the law.

Published in the U.S. by
ULYSSES PRESS
P.O. Box 3440
Berkeley, CA 94703
www.ulyssespress.com

ISBN: 978-1-61243-446-9
Library of Congress Control Number 2014952006

10 9 8 7 6 5 4 3 2 1

Printed in Canada by Marquis Book Printing

Acquisitions Editor: Casie Vogel
Managing Editor: Claire Chun
Editor: Renee Rutledge
Proofreader: Lauren Harrison
Layout: Lindsay Tamura
Indexer: Sayre Van Young
Interior design: what!design @ whatweb.com
Front cover design: Rebecca Lown
Cover photos: © Kate Bello

Distributed by Publishers Group West

NOTE TO READERS: This book has been written and published strictly for informational and educational purposes only. It is not intended to serve as medical advice or to be any form of medical treatment. You should always consult your physician before altering or changing any aspect of your medical treatment and/or undertaking a diet regimen, including the guidelines as described in this book. Do not stop or change any prescription medications without the guidance and advice of your physician. Any use of the information in this book is made on the reader's good judgment after consulting with his or her physician and is the reader's sole responsibility. This book is not intended to diagnose or treat any medical condition and is not a substitute for a physician.

CONTENTS

Introduction 9

Chapter 1   The Benefits of Bath Salts 12

Chapter 2   The Benefits of Essential Oils 16

Chapter 3   Additional Ingredients 18

Chapter 4   How to Make Them 21

Chapter 5   Ailments 26

    Allergy Baths 27

    Baths for Asthma Relief 28

    Baths for Athlete's Foot 29

    Respiratory Baths 30

    Cystic Fibrosis Baths 38

    Calming Baths 39

    Fever-Reducing Baths 42

    Baths for Headaches 43

    Healthy Heart Baths 45

    Anti-Inflammation Baths 46

    Pain-Relieving Baths 47

    Skin-Soothing Baths 54

    Uplifting Baths 56

    Infection-Fighting Baths 58

    Baths for Other Ailments 61

Chapter 6   Skin and Beauty 64

    Acne Baths 65

    Antiaging Baths 66

    Skin-Balancing Baths 68

    Cellulite Baths 69

    Cleansing Baths...70
    Baths for Dry Skin..72
    Oily Skin Baths...77
    Sensitive Skin Baths..79
    Skin-Smoothing Baths..80

Chapter 7   Meditative Baths...............................81
    Salt Soaks..83
    Bath Bombs..88
    Salt Scrubs...91

Chapter 8   Chakras..93
    The Base Chakra...94
    The Sacral Chakra...95
    The Solar Plexus Chakra.....................................97
    The Heart Chakra..98
    The Throat Chakra..100
    The Brow Chakra..101
    The Crown Chakra...103
    The Aura Chakra..104

Chapter 9   Astrology.....................................106
    Aries (March 21 to April 19)...............................107
    Taurus (April 20 to May 20)................................108
    Gemini (May 21 to June 20).................................110
    Cancer (June 22 to July 22)................................111
    Leo (July 23 to August 22).................................113
    Virgo (August 23 to September 21)..........................114
    Libra (September 22 to October 23).........................116
    Scorpio (October 24 to November 21)........................117
    Sagittarius (November 22 to December 21)...................119
    Capricorn (December 22 to January 19)......................120
    Aquarius (January 20 to February 18).......................122
    Pisces (February 19 to March 20)...........................123

Chapter 10   Aphrodisiac Baths 125
    Rose 126
    Jasmine. 127
    Patchouli. 128
    Bergamot. 129

Chapter 11   Bath Recipes for Pregnancy 130

Chapter 12   Bath Blends for Him 135
    Salt Soaks 136
    Salt Scrubs 137
    Bath Bombs. 138

Chapter 13   Seasonal Baths 140
    Winter. 140
    Spring. 144
    Summer 147
    Fall 150

Chapter 14   Floral Baths 154
    Salt Soaks 154
    Salt Scrubs 157
    Bath Bombs. 159

Chapter 15   Baths from Around the World 163

Conclusion 167

Conversions 169

Index 171

Recipe Index. 176

Acknowledgments. 181

About the Author 183

INTRODUCTION

My journey to natural beauty has been a long one. However, I wouldn't have it any other way. Over the years, I've learned so much and debunked many detrimental myths. I think many of us are in the same boat, reading beauty magazines then spending gobs of money on products that don't really work or benefit us in any way.

Now, at 35, I realize that beauty goes hand in hand with mind, body, and spirit. That's why, when I decided to write this book, I wanted to include how natural bath salt soaks affect our overall health.

Let's go back to the beginning. At 19, I was your typical teenager eating fast food, barely working out, and basically doing nothing to improve my overall health. Soon after starting my freshman year of college, I had to drop out after getting sick and being bedridden for over a month. My cholesterol was charted at 270! My doctor could not figure out what was wrong with me, but today I can tell you that my body just gave up on me because I treated it so badly. I had no idea my illness was due to a poor diet, because I hadn't gained any weight. At that young age, I thought I was somehow immune to severe illnesses and could live my life without consequences. Before getting sick, I wasn't paying attention to my body's warning signs: bad skin, fatigue, and catching colds frequently.

It wasn't until I was 27 that I truly became serious about health and natural beauty. I had begun to eat healthier than I had when I was a teenager; however, I still didn't understand what being healthy really meant. I still drank and ate fast food on a semi-regular basis. A drugstore beauty junkie, I was always on the lookout for the next best product that could fix my skin. By my mid-twenties, my acne was gone, but my skin was either very oily or very dry, never balanced. I spent way too much money on products, hoping I could find one I could stick with in the long run that actually lived up to its advertised potential. It never happened.

Then one day, and I can't remember why I did this, I began to look at the ingredients on the back of the bottle. The thought crossed my mind that all of those incomprehensible technical terms couldn't be good for my skin. It was a gut reaction to do a little research.

This was back in 2007, when there wasn't much on the Internet except for the Environmental Working Group's Skin Deep Cosmetics Database, a site dedicated to safe beauty products. And there definitely wasn't a homemade natural beauty movement like there is today. But what I did find in my research is that next to no regulations exist in regard to the ingredients used in beauty products in the United States. And that scared me.

Almost immediately, I decided to ditch my constant search for the magical drugstore product and look into pure natural ingredients from nature. I think there had always been a side to me that wanted to look toward what Mother Earth provides, but before 2007, I would always get sidetracked along the way, distracted by marketing and wanting to fit in. Now my gut was telling me it was time to take the plunge.

The first thing I started was to wash my face with honey. I had read in various places that honey has been used as a beauty product since ancient times, and that it is antiviral and antibacterial, yet extremely gentle. I tried it and it worked! After that, I dove deeper into natural beauty and eventually made my own beauty products. I noticed that my skin began to balance itself out. Now, I can look back and see that it's no coincidence this happened. In addition to completely converting to organic beauty ingredients, I became obsessed with eating as naturally as possible and trying to live an overall healthy lifestyle. Today, I'm a million light-years away from how I lived my life as a teenager, or even in my early 20s. I look better at 35 than I did at 19, and I feel a gazillion times better too.

You may be wondering what this has to do with bath salt soaks. Well, to me it all goes hand in hand. Bath salt soaks are a way to cherish your body. It's almost a sacred practice. When you treat your body as a temple, it will reward you, hands down. Our bodies work extremely hard for us, and relaxing in a natural bath salt soak is a way of giving back.

In this book you will find personalized recipes catered to you and what your body needs physically, emotionally, and mentally. The "Ailments" chapter (page 26) features bath recipes to help relieve everything from flu symptoms to sore muscles. "Skin and Beauty" (page 64) is broken up into baths according to skin types and problem areas, as well as antiaging soaks. Then we'll focus on meditative baths (page 81), baths to open your chakras (page 93), baths based on your astrology sign (page 106), and aphrodisiac baths (page 125). "Bath Recipes for Pregnancy" (page 130), "Bath Blends for Him" (page 135), "Seasonal Baths" (page 140), "Floral Baths" (page 154), and "Baths from Around the World" (page 163) follow.

While you soak delightedly in one of these handcrafted recipes, remember that you're not only easing your muscles and pampering your skin, but allowing your mind to relax and flow in meditation, something that we truly need in today's busy age. I hope you find this helpful in your daily life to keep you grounded, relaxed, content, and happy.

CHAPTER 1
THE BENEFITS OF BATH SALTS

In this book, we will uncover the various reasons for taking baths, from healing and relaxation to beautifying and enjoyment. While we cover a lot of ground, a common theme with every recipe is to promote feeling better in some way or another.

These recipes are one part of a bigger equation. I truly believe that in order to feel our best, we must be balanced in all parts of our lives. Our lifestyles, from the way we eat to our mental attitude, combined with healing rituals like bathing, lead to the results we seek. A healing bath with salts and essential oils is one more piece to completing the puzzle of well-being.

One thing that I've learned is the power of intention. I was already studying how intention works (and watching it work magic in my own life) when I read in Patricia Davis's book, *Subtle Aromatherapy*, about the use of intention when using essential oils. I truly believe setting an intention, especially when it comes to healing, is very powerful.

So, what is the best way to take a bath? It may seem like a funny question, but there is an art to getting the most out of your healing bath. Luckily, it's very simple.

Take your bath at a time when you won't be bothered. There is almost nothing more enjoyable than a luxurious bath at the end of a stressful day. Dim the lights and light a candle. Take the bath in silence or with music that speaks to you. Draw a medium-hot bath and fill the tub, then add your salt soak or bath bomb. Once you're comfortable in the bath, close your eyes and set your intention (details on page 82). Be grateful that you have the luxury of taking a healing bath. Then relax and let the salts and oils do their magic.

Baths Promote Well-Being

Throughout history, salt soaks have been used as a way to heal. Starting in Ancient China and then spreading west to Ancient Egypt, Greece, and Rome, bath salts have been used not only to heal ailments, but also to stay and look youthful. There have even been recent studies that show Dead Sea salts are beneficial in reducing wrinkles.

Because of the high density of minerals in bath salts, such as bromide, calcium, magnesium, potassium, and sodium, soaking in them detoxifies your body while softening and plumping up your skin. Salt soaks have been proven to reduce common skin conditions such as itching, psoriasis, and eczema. Another major benefit of salt soaks is easing sore muscles and tendinitis.

The relaxation of soaking in a tub of hot water and salts reduces stress, which is linked to most diseases and ailments, including the skin conditions listed above. When we are stressed, the immune system is lowered in order for the body to deal with the stress. In other words, we go into fight-or-flight mode, which cuts off our ability to heal ourselves.

These days, stress is a massive part of daily life. Even little things can set it off: checking email, traffic, and everyday busyness. Most of us live in a state of being overwhelmed, especially with the constant use of technology. I'd go as far as to say that in some ways, we are addicted to the feeling of being in fight-or-flight mode. The constant need to be in the know, to be connected, and to be updated leaves us feeling completely exhausted. In fact, there is an actual term for this: adrenal fatigue.

We all deal with adrenal fatigue, whether it is stress from work or the excitement and enthusiasm behind new projects. Adrenal fatigue is not something that should be taken lightly. It ages us and leaves us susceptible to disease. Reducing adrenal overload depends on how we react to the stressors of daily life. Habits we create, such as good nutrition and exercise are key, but meditation is just as important when it comes to overall health. We can't go full throttle all the time. There need to be moments throughout the day where we can turn it off. Slowing things down, being in the moment, and being grounded has done wonders for reducing my own adrenal fatigue. However, this habit takes practice and isn't accomplished overnight.

With a meditative bath (page 81), you can ease your mind and just be, and that is very powerful. Think back to when you had your last relaxing bath. How did you feel before you got in? What was on your mind? Were you stressed thinking about all of the things you needed to do or didn't get done that day? Now how did you feel when you got out? I bet you felt completely at ease and were no longer thinking about your to-do list. The benefits of bath soaks would have worked their magic, and your body would have thanked you for the healing and rejuvenation.

My frame of mind is to treat your body as a temple every day. Healing baths are special, and yes, they feel like a luxury. Baths alone, without an emphasis on well-being through nutrition and lifestyle, are not nearly as powerful. I urge you to use this book as either an addition to your healthy lifestyle or a starting point for an overall balanced way of life. Trust me, it works!

To help make bath salt soaks a regular part of your routine, here are four categories of salts used in the recipes of this book, along with their cleansing qualities:

Coarse Sea Salts   Sea salts have been used for thousands of years for therapeutic baths. Filled with minerals, these salts are used to detoxify the skin and increase circulation while leaving skin soft. Sea salts can come in either fine or coarse grinds. I added coarse sea salts in recipes throughout the books for more texture; however, feel free to switch them out for the fine grind if you prefer.

Dead Sea Salts   Dead Sea salts come directly from the Dead Sea and have a higher salt content than other salts. They are abundant with minerals as well. The healing properties of Dead Sea salts reduce insomnia and anxiety, soothe the skin, relieve muscle ailments, regulate water retention, and detoxify the skin, along with many other therapeutic benefits.

Himalayan Salts   With over 84 minerals, Himalayan salts are among the purest around, known for their beautifying benefits such as combating dry skin, skin ailments, and aging. They also contain some of the same benefits as Dead Sea salts, such as regulating water retention, reducing sleep disorders, and calming nerves.

Epsom Salts   Containing mainly magnesium sulfate, Epsom salts are known for easing muscle soreness and joint pain. Their cleansing properties combat oily skin. If you're on a budget, switch the Dead Sea or Himalayan varieties for Epsom salts, the most reasonably priced of the three.

CHAPTER 2
THE BENEFITS OF ESSENTIAL OILS

Essential oils are magical. Their scents and properties link us back to what Mother Earth intended to nurture us with: plants. As you make the recipes in this book, you'll find each oil and its corresponding scent evokes something different. This could be memories, feelings, or a sense of well-being.

One of the most enjoyable aspects of creating these recipes was coming up with combinations based on the scents I was drawn to and figuring out what they reminded me of. Benzoin is like warm chocolate. Bergamot is a walk through Rome. Eucalyptus feels like clarity and rejuvenation. Rose is romance. Jasmine is femininity. The list goes on and on.

As a self-declared health nut, learning about different properties of essential oils and which work well for certain ailments is fascinating. I love learning about home remedies and ways to heal myself.

As with bath salts, essential oils are more powerful when combined with a healthy lifestyle. That's when the real transformation begins and you will find that a little bit of these special oils goes a long way.

When it comes to buying oils, use discretion. Many companies sell low-quality, diluted oils. Be picky. There is no point spending money on oil that doesn't contain the properties you're looking for. I bought most of my oils from Mountain Rose Herbs at MountainRoseHerbs.com. I absolutely love this company and have been using them for years. Buy organic if you can; however, not all oils are available organic. If that is the case, be sure to buy pesticide-free or wild-grown oils. All oils at Mountain Rose Herbs are pesticide-free, even if they're not organic.

Baths are almost the perfect way to utilize the benefits of essential oils, especially when combined with salts. The salts ease sore muscles, soften the skin, and detoxify, while each essential oil has different healing properties for specific ailments, skin issues, and even emotional stress, as you will see in the following chapters.

Take Precautions

Essential oils are very strong and powerful. Pregnant women should check with their doctor before using essential oils because some can be quite dangerous. That also goes for babies, children, and the elderly. For any of these age groups, the amount of oils in these recipes should be cut in half to be on the safe side.

Here is a list of essential oils that are okay to use during pregnancy:

- Neroli
- Mandarin
- Rose (after the first trimester)
- Lavender (after the first trimester)
- Roman Chamomile (after the first trimester)

CHAPTER 3
ADDITIONAL INGREDIENTS

In addition to salts and essential oils, there are some other ingredients that are needed mainly for making salt scrubs, salt soaks, and bath bombs.

Carrier Oils

Organic vegetable carrier oils are a must-have for any homemade skincare regimen. In this book they are used mainly for salt scrubs, but I also love to use them instead of lotion after a bath or shower. Store in a dark, cool, and dry area when not in use.

Almond Oil Almond oil is a great base for salt scrubs because of its sweet smell and lighter consistency. It is commonly used in beauty products because of its ability to moisturize skin.

Avocado Oil Avocado oil is perfect for those with dry or mature skin because of its extremely rich consistency and blend of vitamins.

Coconut Oil   One of the most widely used oils today for beauty products and cooking, coconut oil is extremely rich with a light coconut scent. One of my go-to oils for everyday use.

Jojoba Oil   This is a great oil for those with acne and oily skin because of its light and easily absorbable consistency.

Kukui Nut Oil   The kukui nut, hailing from the Hawaiian islands, creates a luxurious and rich oil that easily absorbs into the skin.

Olive Oil   Olive oil is one of the most widely used oils for skincare products because of its moisturizing ability.

Rosehip Oil   Considered one of the best carrier oils for antiaging, rosehip oil is used for reducing wrinkles and scars. Rosehip seed oil is rich in essential fatty acids yet very easily absorbed into the skin.

Sesame Oil   An all-around versatile oil used in cooking and skincare products, sesame oil is rich and moisturizing. It is widely used in Ayurveda for its antibacterial and anti-inflammatory properties.

Sunflower Oil   Great oil for beauty products because of its vitamin A, D, and E content and rich consistency, sunflower oil also has next to no scent, perfect for mixing with essential oils.

Clays

Clays are used in salt soaks to draw out impurities and soften the skin. They're great for all skin types, but those who are oily or acne-prone may benefit the most since the clays soak up excessive oil from the skin. I purchase my clays from Mountain Rose Herbs, although they're rather easy to find online from other vendors as well.

French Green Clay   French green clay tones and revitalizes skin by drawing out impurities and tightening pores.

Fuller's Earth Clay This is considered the best clay for oily and acne-prone skin because of its oil-drawing capabilities.

Rhassoul Clay This Moroccan clay is filled with minerals such as calcium, iron, magnesium, and potassium.

Additional Ingredients

Both baking soda and citric acid are must-have ingredients for bath bombs.

Baking Soda This is used in bath bombs for its cleansing and deodorizing properties.

Citric Acid Found mainly in lemons and limes, citric acid is used in bath bombs to create the fizzing effect.

CHAPTER 4
HOW TO MAKE THEM

The best things are the simplest things, especially when it comes to health and beauty. In this book you will find an array of recipes for salts soaks, salt scrubs, and bath bombs. Making these simple creations brings together all aspects of our life: health, beauty, love, travel, and spirituality.

Salt Soaks

Salt soaks are a simple way to give your body the extra love and attention it needs. Salt soaks are a combination of salt, essential oils, and sometimes beautifying and detoxifying clays. They are extremely therapeutic and can be used to heal a number of different ailments or skin issues. They are probably best known as being used for relaxation after a long day or used to reduce stress. As you will see with the array of different types of salt soaks, their uses are almost endless.

SUPPLIES

- Mixing bowl
- Measuring cups
- Measuring spoons
- 26-ounce to 32-ounce glass jar for storage (depending on recipe)
- Whisk (optional)

STORAGE

As far as storing the bath salts, it's entirely up to you to decide how fancy you would like to get. I do recommend storing the salts in a glass container or jar. Glass mason jars work great, plus their pricing is extremely reasonable. You can find more decorative jars at a local craft store or my favorite place to buy most of my online ingredients, Mountain Rose Herbs.

> ### Sterilize Your Storage Jar
>
> Be sure to always sterilize any jar or container you use for a homemade beauty recipe. The process is very easy. Bring a large pot of water to a boil and then let the glass jar or container simmer in the boiling water for about five minutes. Remove and place on a clean towel to dry and cool off. This will ensure that you're putting your salt soak into a clean container and will help it stay fresh longer.

DIRECTIONS

For all the salt soak recipes in this book, follow these directions. You'll find that creating different salt soaks is just a matter of switching up the ingredients for the desired outcome.

1. Measure out and add the dry ingredients to a mixing bowl.
2. Mix your dry ingredients with clean hands or a whisk if you prefer.
3. Add oils and mix again.

4. Pour mixture (you may want to use a spoon for this) into a jar.

5. Store in a cool, dry, and dark area when not in use.

Salt Scrubs

Salt scrubs are mainly used to remove dead and dry skin. You will find your skin literally glowing after using them! They are also great for reenergizing and leave you feeling invigorated. You can use salt scrubs in a shower or before soaking in a bath.

SUPPLIES

- Measuring cups
- Measuring spoons
- Small spoon for mixing
- 250-ml mason jar for storage

STORAGE

I usually use smaller mason jars for scrubs. Scrubs can last up to a month or so, but longer than that is not recommended. Vitamin E oil can be added to the recipes as a preservative.

DIRECTIONS

As with the salt soaks, making a scrub is one of the easiest things you will ever do. So worth the reward it hardly seems possible that something this simple works wonders when it comes to your overall health and beauty. Scrubs will leave your skin glowing and help reduce stress, vital for overall wellness.

Follow this set of directions for all of the salt scrub recipes, switching out the ingredients depending on the recipe.

1. Sterilize your storage jar (page 22).

2. After the jar has dried and cooled, add salt to the jar.

3. Add vegetable/nut carrier oil and mix.

4. Add essential oils and mix thoroughly.

5. Store in a dark, cool, and dry area when not in use.

Bath Bombs

Unlike salt soaks, bath bombs are actually dry, molded mixtures of salts, clays, baking soda, citric acid, and essential oils that fizz when you drop them in water.

Here is where we get scientific. Where measuring for salt soaks and scrubs is not exactly crucial, it is for bath bombs. It took me some experimenting to get my first bath bombs to work, but then they were buzzing and fizzing like no other. It was really exciting! These make great gifts, as there's something really playful about them. They also have similar benefits to salt soaks. They're extremely relaxing after the fizzing has subsided; many are included as alternative options to the soaks in this book.

Because these are natural bath bombs, there is no added food coloring in these recipes. If you're trying to switch over to natural beauty, the last thing you want to do is soak in a bath full of toxins. So instead, I added floral powders to some of the recipes for coloring. These powders also contain benefits similar to essential oils.

SUPPLIES

- Mold for bath bomb (molds can be found on Amazon, eBay, and Etsy, or use a cookie mold from your local kitchen supply)
- Two bowls
- Whisk

STORAGE

As far as storage goes, the same mason jars you would use for the salt soaks work well. Choose a larger size for the bath bombs.

DIRECTIONS

For all of the bath bomb recipes in this book, follow this set of directions and switch out the ingredients depending on the recipe.

1. Mix dry ingredients together.
2. In a separate bowl, mix water, coconut or carrier oil, and essential oil.
3. Pour the liquid a little bit at a time into the dry ingredients and mix.
4. After the mixture begins to clump together, fill the mold as much as possible, as this will help hold it together. (You may not need to use all of the liquid if the mixture is already clumping.)
5. Once the mold is formed, just tap out the bath bomb and let it dry for 12 to 24 hours (avoid leaving it in a room with humidity).

CHAPTER 5
AILMENTS

Soaking in a bath can help you forget about your aches and pains. Many of these ailments are caused by stress, for which an aromatherapy salt soak is the perfect medicine. Reduce stress and you reduce the likelihood for disease.

In this section you may find two to three recipes for one ailment. This is because there is a wider variety of essential oils that have healing properties for that particular ailment. I grouped the essential oils in each recipe based on how well the scents went together, but feel free to mix and match to your choosing.

Also, be sure to switch out essential oils every three weeks or so. Using the same essential oil every day can be toxic for your body. For those ailments that only have one recipe, take some time off between baths or take a relaxing bath with different essential oils in between.

For more information about using essential oils to combat ailments, I highly recommend the book *Aromatherapy: An A-Z* by Patricia Davis. Packed with great detailed information, it's my go-to handbook for any time I'm feeling under the weather.

Allergy Baths

Seasonal allergies or hay fever tend to come on under stress; these soaks are ideal for allergy prevention.

Allergy Salt Soak 1

2 cups of Dead Sea salts
1 cup of Epsom salts
½ cup of baking soda
5 drops of jasmine essential oil
5 drops of sandalwood essential oil

Allergy Salt Soak 2

2 cups of Dead Sea salts
1 cup of Epsom salts
½ cup of baking soda
5 drops of bergamot essential oil
5 drops of clary sage essential oil

Allergy Salt Soak 3

2 cups of Dead Sea salts
1 cup of Epsom salts
½ cup of baking soda
5 drops of rose essential oil
5 drops of neroli essential oil

Allergy Salt Soak 4

2 cups of Dead Sea salts

1 cup of Epsom salts

½ cup of baking soda

10 drops of chamomile essential oil

Baths for Asthma Relief

Asthma Salt Soak to Relieve or Prevent Spasms 1

2 cups of Dead Sea salts

1 cup of Epsom salts

½ cup of baking soda

5 drops of chamomile essential oil

5 drops of rose essential oil

Asthma Salt Soak to Relieve or Prevent Spasms 2

2 cups of Himalayan salts

1 cup of coarse sea salts

½ cup of baking soda

1 cup of rhassoul clay

5 drops of bergamot essential oil

5 drops of lavender essential oil

Asthma Salt Soak to Relieve and Calm Chest Infection

This is soak is also ideal for those without asthma, but who are experiencing chest congestion.

2 cups of Dead Sea salts

1 cup of Epsom salts

½ cup of baking soda

5 drops of frankincense essential oil

5 drops of lavender essential oil

Baths for Athlete's Foot

Clean feet before soaking. After bath, dry feet thoroughly to prevent recurrence of the fungus that causes athlete's foot, which grows in moist conditions.

Athlete's Foot Salt Soak 1

2 cups of Dead Sea salts

1 cup of Epsom salts

½ cup of baking soda

5 drops of lavender essential oil

5 drops of myrrh essential oil

Athlete's Foot Salt Soak 2

2 cups of Dead Sea salts

1 cup of Epsom salts

½ cup of baking soda

10 drops of tea tree essential oil

Respiratory Baths

Use the following soaks at the first sign of respiratory infection as well as during infection to help speed up recovery.

Respiratory Salt Soak 1

1 cup of Dead Sea salts

1 cup of Epsom salts

1 cup of coarse sea salts

½ cup of baking soda

1 cup of French green clay

5 drops of eucalyptus essential oil

5 drops of peppermint essential oil

Respiratory Salt Soak 2

1 cup of Dead Sea salts

1 cup of Epsom salts

1 cup of coarse sea salts

½ cup of baking soda

5 drops of bergamot essential oil

5 drops of lavender essential oil

Respiratory Salt Soak 3

1 cup of Dead Sea salts

2 cups of Epsom salts

½ cup of baking soda

10 drops of basil essential oil

Disinfectant Salt Soak for Cold and Flu Prevention

Use the following recipe after being exposed or at the first sign of cold or flu.

2 cups of Dead Sea salts

1 cup of Epsom salts

½ cup of baking soda

5 drops of tea tree essential oil

5 drops of eucalyptus essential oil

5 drops of bergamot essential oil

Congestion Salt Soak

Use the following salt soak to minimize congestion due to pollen and other allergens.

1 cup of Dead Sea salts

1 cup of Epsom salts

1 cup of coarse sea salts

½ cup of baking soda

1 cup of French green clay

5 drops of lavender essential oil

5 drops of chamomile essential oil

Dry coughs can be caused by dry air, dust, allergies, or viruses. They don't produce phlegm; rather it's a sign that your airways are irritated. The following recipes are meant to clear out irritants and relieve airways.

Bronchitis Salt Soak for Dry Cough 1

1 cup of Dead Sea salts

1 cup of Epsom salts

1 cup of coarse sea salts

½ cup of baking soda

5 drops of bergamot essential oil

5 drops of eucalyptus essential oil

Bronchitis Salt Soak for Dry Cough 2

2 cups of Dead Sea salts

1 cup of Epsom salts

½ cup of baking soda

5 drops of lavender essential oil

5 drops of sandalwood essential oil

Bronchitis Salt Soak for Dry Cough 3

1 cup of Dead Sea salts

1 cup of Epsom salts

1 cup of coarse sea salts

½ cup of baking soda

10 drops of benzoin essential oil

Use the following soaks at the first sign of chest congestion to help stop it in its tracks.

Cold and Flu Congestion Salt Soak 1

1 cup of Dead Sea salts

1 cup of Epsom salts

1 cup of coarse sea salts

½ cup of baking soda

5 drops of eucalyptus essential oil

5 drops of tea tree essential oil

Cold and Flu Congestion Salt Soak 2

1 cup of Dead Sea salts

1 cup of Epsom salts

1 cup of coarse sea salts

½ cup of baking soda

10 drops of peppermint essential oil

Cold and Flu Congestion Salt Soak 3

1 cup of Dead Sea salts

1 cup of Epsom salts

1 cup of coarse sea salts

½ cup of baking soda

10 drops of lavender essential oil

It's best to take a bath at the first sign of infection. Go straight to bed after bathing. If you develop a full-blown flu, repeat the bath over the next two to three days.

Influenza Salt Soak 1

1 cup of Dead Sea salts
1 cup of Epsom salts
1 cup of coarse sea salts
½ cup of baking soda
5 drops of eucalyptus essential oil
5 drops of lavender essential oil

Influenza Salt Soak 2

1 cup of Dead Sea salts
1 cup of Epsom salts
1 cup of coarse sea salts
½ cup of baking soda
5 drops of tea tree essential oil
5 drops of bergamot essential oil
2 drops of eucalyptus essential oil

The following recipes are ideal for facilitating "productive" coughs during or after a cold or flu. These will help expel mucus that is causing chest congestion.

Salt Soak for Expelling Mucus 1

1 cup of Dead Sea salts
1 cup of Epsom salts
1 cup of coarse sea salts
½ cup of baking soda
5 drops of basil essential oil
5 drops of myrrh essential oil

Salt Soak for Expelling Mucus 2

1 cup of Dead Sea salts
1 cup of Epsom salts
1 cup of coarse sea salts
½ cup of baking soda
5 drops of benzoin essential oil
5 drops of myrrh essential oil
5 drops of frankincense essential oil

Using these recipes at the first sign of a cold will oftentimes stop it right in its tracks. They could be used as a preventive measure if you've been exposed to a cold or it's cold/flu season.

Common Cold Salt Soak 1

1 cup of Dead Sea salts
1 cup of Epsom salts
1 cup of coarse sea salts
½ cup of baking soda
5 drops of tea tree essential oil
5 drops of eucalyptus essential oil
2 drops of lavender essential oil

Common Cold Salt Soak 2

1 cup of Dead Sea salts
1 cup of Epsom salts
1 cup of coarse sea salts
½ cup of baking soda
10 drops of lavender essential oil

Common Cold Salt Soak 3

2 cups of Dead Sea salts
1 cup of Epsom salts
½ cup of baking soda
10 drops of tea tree essential oil

Common Cold Salt Soak 4

Use this particular salt soak to reduce the shivers.

1 cup of Epsom salts
1 cup of Dead Sea salts
1 cup of coarse sea salts
½ cup of baking soda
10 drops of marjoram essential oil

Common Cold Salt Soak 5

This one's an evening soak for cold prevention.

2 cups of Dead Sea salts
1 cup of Epsom salts
½ cup of baking soda
5 drops of lavender essential oil
5 drops of marjoram essential oil

Cystic Fibrosis Baths

Cystic fibrosis is a genetic disorder. The following soaks can be used for relief; however, see your doctor if you have serious symptoms, as this can be a life-threatening illness.

Cystic Fibrosis Salt Soak 1

1 cup of Dead Sea salts
1 cup of Epsom salts
1 cup of coarse sea salts
½ cup of baking soda
5 drops of frankincense essential oil
5 drops of lavender essential oil
2 drops of eucalyptus essential oil

Cystic Fibrosis Salt Soak 2

1 cup of Dead Sea salts
1 cup of Epsom salts
1 cup of coarse sea salts
½ cup of baking soda
5 drops of myrrh essential oil
5 drops of benzoin essential oil
2 drops of tea tree essential oil

Cystic Fibrosis Salt Soak 3

1 cup of Dead Sea salts

1 cup of Epsom salts

1 cup of coarse sea salts

½ cup of baking soda

5 drops of ravensara essential oil

5 drops of sandalwood essential oil

Calming Baths

De-stress Salt Soak 1

2 cups of Himalayan salts

1 cup of coarse sea salts

½ cup of baking soda

1 cup of fuller's earth clay

5 drops of neroli essential oil

5 drops of rose essential oil

2 drops of marjoram essential oil

De-stress Salt Soak 2

2 cups of Himalayan salts

1 cup of coarse sea salts

½ cup of baking soda

5 drops of lavender essential oil

5 drops of chamomile essential oil

De-stress Bath Bomb

3 tablespoons of citric acid

2 tablespoons of baking soda

2 tablespoons of cornstarch

2 tablespoons of Epsom salts

1 tablespoon of water

¼ tablespoon of coconut oil

10 drops of jasmine essential oil

De-stress Salt Scrub

1 cup of Dead Sea Salts

¼ cup of almond oil

¼ cup of sunflower oil

3 drops of bergamot essential oil

3 drops of chamomile essential oil

2 drops of lavender essential oil

Calming Salt Soak 1

2 cups of Dead Sea salts

1 cup of Himalayan salts

½ cup of baking soda

1 cup of French green clay

5 drops of chamomile essential oil

5 drops of lavender essential oil

2 drops of rose essential oil

Calming Salt Soak 2

2 cups of Dead Sea salts
1 cup of Epsom salts
½ cup of baking soda
5 drops of jasmine essential oil
5 drops of sandalwood essential oil

Calming Salt Soak 3

Bergamot is calming, yet is considered somewhat invigorating and uplifting as well.

1 cup of Dead Sea salts
1 cup of Epsom salts
1 cup of coarse sea salts
½ cup of baking soda
1 cup of French green clay
10 drops of bergamot essential oil

Fever-Reducing Baths

Use the following salt soaks at the first sign of fever to stop it in its tracks or to the break fever. Prepare a lukewarm bath instead of hot.

Fever-Reducing Salt Soak 1

2 cups of Epsom salts

1 cup of Dead Sea salts

½ cup of baking soda

5 drops of birch (black or yellow) essential oil

5 drops of peppermint essential oil

Fever-Reducing Salt Soak 2

1 cup of Dead Sea salts

1 cup of Epsom salts

1 cup of coarse sea salts

½ cup of baking soda

5 drops of basil essential oil

5 drops of chamomile essential oil

Fever-Reducing Salt Soak 3

1 cup of Dead Sea salts

1 cup of Epsom salts

1 cup of coarse sea salts

½ cup of baking soda

5 drops of lavender essential oil

5 drops of tea tree essential oil

Fever-Reducing Salt Soak 4

1 cup of Dead Sea salts

1 cup of Epsom salts

1 cup of coarse sea salts

½ cup of baking soda

10 drops of peppermint essential oil

Baths for Headaches

Many essential oils are great for relieving headaches. I've created five different baths for this ailment because I've found that the simpler the scent, the more effective the bath is for reducing headaches. Too many scents combined can actually worsen a headache.

Headache Salt Soak 1

2 cups of Himalayan salts

1 cup of coarse sea salts

½ cup of baking soda

10 drops of lavender essential oil

Headache Salt Soak 2

2 cups of Dead Sea salts

1 cup of Epsom salts

½ cup of baking soda

10 drops of peppermint essential oil

Ailments

Headache Salt Soak 3

2 cups of Dead Sea salts

1 cup of Epsom salts

½ cup of baking soda

10 drops of rosemary essential oil

Headache Salt Soak 4

2 cups of Himalayan salts

1 cup of coarse sea salts

½ cup of baking soda

1 cup of fuller's earth clay

5 drops of lavender essential oil

5 drops of bergamot essential oil

Headache Salt Soak 5

For headache caused by sinus infection.

1 cup of Dead Sea salts

1 cup of Epsom salts

1 cup of coarse sea salts

½ cup of baking soda

1 cup of French green clay

10 drops of eucalyptus essential oil

Healthy Heart Baths

High Blood Pressure Salt Soak

2 cups of Dead Sea salts

1 cup of Himalayan salts

½ cup of baking soda

5 drops of lavender essential oil

5 drops of bergamot essential oil

Low Blood Pressure Salt Soak

Use sparingly.

2 cups of Dead Sea salts

1 cup of Epsom salts

½ cup of baking soda

10 drops of peppermint essential oil

For a rapid heartbeat after a stressful situation.

Tachycardia Salt Soak 1

2 cups of Dead Sea salts

1 cup of Epsom salts

½ cup of baking soda

5 drops of ylang-ylang essential oil

5 drops of chamomile essential oil

Tachycardia Salt Soak 2

2 cups of Himalayan salts

1 cup of coarse sea salts

½ cup of baking soda

5 drops of lavender essential oil

5 drops of neroli essential oil

5 drops of rose essential oil

Anti-Inflammation Baths

Anti-Inflammation Salt Soak

Chamomile and lavender essential oils work well for reducing inflammation.

2 cups of Himalayan salts

1 cup of coarse sea salts

½ cup of baking soda

1 cup of fuller's earth clay

5 drops of chamomile essential oil

5 drops of lavender essential oil

Tendinitis Salt Soak

Tendinitis is a form of inflammation. Switch out this bath with the Anti-Inflammation Salt Soak every three weeks for chronic tendinitis.

- **1** cup of Dead Sea salts
- **1** cup of Epsom salts
- **1** cup of coarse sea salts
- **½** cup of baking soda
- **5** drops of birch (black or yellow) essential oil
- **5** drops of peppermint essential oil

Pain-Relieving Baths

Dull Aches and Pains Salt Soak

- **2** cups of Himalayan salts
- **1** cup of coarse sea salts
- **½** cup of baking soda
- **10** drops of chamomile essential oil

Sharp Aches and Pains Salt Soak

- **2** cups of Himalayan salts
- **1** cup of coarse sea salts
- **½** cup of baking soda
- **10** drops of lavender essential oil

Muscle Pain Salt Soak

1 cup of Dead Sea salts

2 cups of Epsom salts

½ cup of baking soda

5 drops of marjoram essential oil

5 drops of lavender essential oil

Muscle Relaxer Salt Soak

2 cups of Epsom salts

1 cup of Himalayan salts

½ cup of baking soda

10 drops of jasmine essential oil

Repetitive Strain Injury Salt Soak

If you have a repetitive strain injury, switch this soak out every three weeks with either the Muscle Pain Salt Soak or Muscle Relaxer Salt Soak.

1 cup of Dead Sea salts

2 cups of Epsom salts

½ cup of baking soda

10 drops of birch essential oil

Backache Salt Soak for Fatigue, Spasm, or Tension 1

1 cup of Dead Sea salts

2 cups of Epsom salts

½ cup of baking soda

5 drops of lavender essential oil

5 drops of marjoram essential oil

Backache Salt Soak for Fatigue, Spasm, or Tension 2

1 cup of Dead Sea salts

2 cups of Epsom salts

½ cup of baking soda

10 drops of rosemary essential oil

Sciatica Salt Soak

Use the Sciatica Salt Soak to combat pain along the sciatic nerve in the legs.

2 cups of Himalayan salts

1 cup of coarse sea salts

½ cup of baking soda

1 cup of rhassoul clay

10 drops of chamomile essential oil

Muscle spasms are often times symptoms of arthritis.

Detoxifying Arthritis Salt Soak

Loosen up joints with this detoxifying salt soak. It is ideal to move around a bit after your bath to keep joints loose and avoid stiffness.

2 cups of Himalayan salts
1 cup of coarse sea salts
½ cup of baking soda
1 cup of rhassoul clay
5 drops of lemon grass essential oil
5 drops of cypress essential oil

Arthritis Salt Soak for Circulation

In some cases arthritis can be caused by poor circulation rather than injury or age. The following recipe uses black pepper essential oil, ideal for getting your blood flowing.

1 cup of Dead Sea salts
1 cup of Epsom salts
1 cup of coarse sea salts
½ cup of baking soda
1 cup of French green clay
5 drops of black pepper essential oil
5 drops of marjoram essential oil

The following Pain-Reducing Arthritis Soak recipes use essential oils ideal for reducing pain rather than loosening joints. However, you may want to switch these out with the previous soak in order to benefit from both. As with the Detoxifying Arthritis Salt Soak, try to move around a bit after your bath to avoid stiffness.

Pain-Reducing Arthritis Salt Soak 1

2 cups of Epsom salts
1 cup of coarse sea salts
½ cup of baking soda
1 cup of rhassoul clay
5 drops of juniper essential oil
5 drops of fennel essential oil
2 drops of benzoin essential oil

Pain-Reducing Arthritis Salt Soak 2

2 cups of Dead Sea salts
1 cup of Epsom salts
½ cup of baking soda
10 drops of lavender essential oil

Pain-Reducing Arthritis Salt Soak 3

2 cups of Dead Sea salts
1 cup of Epsom salts
½ cup of baking soda
10 drops of chamomile essential oil

Heat often helps with cramping, so with these soaks, a hot bath is ideal.

Painful Periods Salt Soak 1

1 cup of Dead Sea salts

1 cup of Epsom salts

1 cup of coarse sea salts

½ cup of baking soda

5 drops of lavender essential oil

5 drops of chamomile essential oil

Painful Periods Salt Soak 2

1 cup of Dead Sea salts

1 cup of Epsom salts

1 cup of coarse sea salts

½ cup of baking soda

10 drops of basil or sweet marjoram essential oil

Use the following salt soaks to reduce depression and irritability.

PMS Salt Soak 1

1 cup of Dead Sea salts

1 cup of Epsom salts

1 cup of coarse sea salts

½ cup of baking soda

10 drops of chamomile essential oil

PMS Salt Soak 2

2 cups of Himalayan salts
1 cup of coarse sea salts
½ cup of baking soda
1 cup of fuller's earth clay
5 drops of rose essential oil
5 drops of lavender essential oil

PMS Salt Soak 3

2 cups of Dead Sea salts
1 cup of Himalayan salts
½ cup of baking soda
1 cup of French green clay
5 drops of bergamot essential oil
5 drops of chamomile essential oil

Skin-Soothing Baths

Salt Soak for Boils

Boils are contagious and can get worse quickly, so it's best to use this soak at the first sign of one.

1 cup of Dead Sea salts
1 cup of Epsom salts
1 cup of coarse sea salts
½ cup of baking soda
1 cup of French green clay
5 drops of juniper essential oil
5 drops of lavender essential oil

Sunburn Salt Soak

When relieving sunburn, prepare a lukewarm bath.

2 cups of Himalayan salts
1 cup of coarse sea salts
½ cup of baking soda
1 cup of fuller's earth clay
10 drops of chamomile essential oil

Soothing Salt Scrub for Itching 1

¾ cup of Dead Sea salts

¼ cup of almond oil

¼ cup of sunflower oil

6 drops of chamomile essential oil

Soothing Salt Scrub for Itching 2

¾ cup of Himalayan salts

¼ cup of almond oil

¼ cup of sunflower oil

6 drops of lavender essential oil

Soothing Salt Soak for Itching

2 cups of Dead Sea salts

1 cup of Himalayan salts

½ cup of baking soda

1 cup of French green clay

10 drops of lavender essential oil

Uplifting Baths

Antidepressant Salt Soak

2 cups of Himalayan salts

1 cup of coarse sea salts

½ cup of baking soda

1 cup of fuller's earth clay

5 drops of bergamot essential oil

5 drops of citronella essential oil

Uplifting Mood Salt Scrub

¾ cup of Dead Sea salts

¼ cup of almond oil

¼ cup of sunflower oil

3 drops of bergamot essential oil

3 drops of orange essential oil

Fatigue Salt Soak

Geranium essential oil relieves fatigue as well acts as an antidepressant for those affected with chronic fatigue.

2 cups of Himalayan salts

1 cup of coarse sea salts

½ cup of baking soda

10 drops of geranium essential oil

Rejuvenating Salt Soak

2 cups of Himalayan salts

1 cup of coarse sea salts

½ cup of baking soda

1 cup of fuller's earth clay

5 drops of jasmine essential oil

5 drops of sandalwood essential oil

Rejuvenating Salt Scrub

¾ cup of Dead Sea salts

¼ cup of almond oil

¼ cup of sunflower oil

6 drops of rose essential oil

• • • • • • • • • • • • • • • •

Both of the following invigorating baths for mental fatigue are used for increased alertness. It should be noted, however, that mental fatigue is best helped by adequate rest and breaks from mental stimulation throughout the day. Use these baths sparingly.

Mental Fatigue Salt Soak

2 cups of Dead Sea salts

1 cup of Epsom salts

½ cup of baking soda

10 drops of basil essential oil

Ailments

Mental Fatigue Salt Scrub

¾ cup of Dead Sea salts

¼ cup of almond oil

¼ cup of sunflower oil

6 drops of peppermint essential oil

Infection-Fighting Baths

Use these recipes at the first sign of infection or after you've been exposed to prevent a full-blown infection.

Antibacterial Salt Soak 1

1 cup of Dead Sea salts

1 cup of Epsom salts

1 cup of coarse sea salts

½ cup of baking soda

1 cup of French green clay

5 drops of lavender essential oil

5 drops of tea tree essential oil

Antibacterial Salt Soak 2

1 cup of Dead Sea salts

1 cup of Epsom salts

1 cup of coarse sea salts

½ cup of baking soda

1 cup of French green clay

10 drops of rosemary essential oil

Lymphatic Cleanse Salt Soak

Use this bath in addition to exercise, drinking plenty of water, and deep breathing to cleanse your lymphatic system.

- **1** cup of Dead Sea salts
- **1** cup of Epsom salts
- **1** cup of coarse sea salts
- **½** cup of baking soda
- **1** cup of French green clay
- **5** drops of rosemary essential oil
- **5** drops of geranium essential oil

Urinary Tract Infection Salt Soak 1

- **1** cup of Dead Sea salts
- **1** cup of Epsom salts
- **1** cup of coarse sea salts
- **½** cup of baking soda
- **5** drops of tea tree essential oil
- **5** drops of sandalwood essential oil

Urinary Tract Infection Salt Soak 2

- **2** cups of Dead Sea salts
- **1** cup of Epsom salts
- **½** cup of baking soda
- **5** drops of bergamot essential oil
- **5** drops of peppermint essential oil

Ailments

Urinary Tract Infection Salt Soak 3

2 cups of Himalayan salts

1 cup of coarse sea salts

½ cup of baking soda

10 drops of chamomile essential oil

. . . .

The following soaks contain essential oils known for being antibacterial, antiviral, and strengthening for your immune system.

Immunity Salt Soak 1

1 cup of Dead Sea salts

1 cup of Epsom salts

1 cup of coarse sea salts

½ cup of baking soda

5 drops of eucalyptus essential oil

5 drops of bergamot essential oil

Immunity Salt Soak 2

2 cups of Dead Sea salts

1 cup of Epsom salts

½ cup of baking soda

5 drops of tea tree essential oil

5 drops of lavender essential oil

Viral Infection Salt Soak 1

1 cup of Dead Sea salts

1 cup of Epsom salts

1 cup of coarse sea salts

½ cup of baking soda

1 cup of French green clay

5 drops of tea tree essential oil

5 drops of bergamot essential oil

Viral Infection Salt Soak 2

2 cups of Dead Sea salts

1 cup of Epsom salts

½ cup of baking soda

5 drops of eucalyptus essential oil

5 drops of lavender essential oil

2 drops of rosemary essential oil

Baths for Other Ailments

Chickenpox Salt Soak 1

1 cup of Dead Sea salts

1 cup of Epsom salts

1 cup of coarse sea salts

½ cup of baking soda

1 cup of French green clay

10 drops of bergamot essential oil

Chickenpox Salt Soak 2

1 cup of Dead Sea salts

1 cup of Epsom salts

1 cup of coarse sea salts

½ cup of baking soda

1 cup of French green clay

5 drops of tea tree essential oil

5 drops of chamomile essential oil

2 drops of lavender essential oil

Hemorrhoids Salt Soak 1

2 cups of Himalayan salts

1 cup of coarse sea salts

½ cup of baking soda

10 drops of frankincense essential oil

Hemorrhoids Salt Soak 2

2 cups of Dead Sea salts

1 cup of Epsom salts

½ cup of baking soda

10 drops of juniper essential oil

Varicose Veins Salt Soak

Extreme heat can actually worsen varicose veins, so prepare a lukewarm bath.

2 cups of Himalayan salts
1 cup of coarse sea salts
½ cup of baking soda
5 drops of cypress essential oil
5 drops of lavender essential oil

Yeast Infection Salt Soak

Use at the first sign of infection or until the infection clears up. If you have a yeast infection, it's also recommended to stay clear of refined sugar and processed foods.

1 cup of Dead Sea salts
1 cup of Epsom salts
1 cup of coarse sea salts
½ cup of baking soda
5 drops of tea tree essential oil
5 drops of lavender essential oil

CHAPTER 6
SKIN AND BEAUTY

It is great to know that nature provides everything you need to stay youthful. With natural beauty remedies, there is no need for creams and pills.

One culprit that affects your health *and* physical appearance? Stress. With elements of nature to help you heal and grow, the following salt soaks, salt scrubs, and bath bombs allow your body to release stress, leaving you glowing.

Acne Baths

Acne Purifying Salt Soak 1

1 cup of Dead Sea salts
1 cup of Epsom salts
1 cup of coarse sea salts
½ cup of baking soda
1 cup of French green clay
5 drops of rosemary essential oil
5 drops of geranium essential oil

Acne Purifying Salt Soak 2

2 cups of Himalayan salts
1 cup of coarse sea salts
½ cup of baking soda
1 cup of fuller's earth clay
5 drops of tea tree essential oil
5 drops of lavender essential oil

Acne Salt Scrub

¾ cup of Himalayan salts
¼ cup of almond oil
¼ cup of kukui nut oil
3 drops of tea tree essential oil
3 drops of lavender essential oil

Skin and Beauty

Acne Bath Bomb

3 tablespoons of citric acid

2 tablespoons of baking soda

2 tablespoons of cornstarch

2 tablespoons of Epsom salts

1 tablespoon of water

¼ tablespoon of coconut oil

10 drops of juniper essential oil

Antiaging Baths

Antiaging Salt Soak 1

2 cups of Himalayan salts

1 cup of coarse sea salts

½ cup of baking soda

1 cup of rhassoul clay

5 drops of frankincense essential oil

5 drops of sandalwood essential oil

Antiaging Salt Soak 2

2 cups of Himalayan salts

1 cup of coarse sea salts

½ cup of baking soda

1 cup of fuller's earth clay

5 drops of carrot seed essential oil

5 drops of bergamot essential oil

Antiaging Salt Soak 3

2 cups of Dead Sea salts

1 cup of Himalayan salts

½ cup of baking soda

1 cup of French green clay

10 drops of rose essential oil

Antiaging Salt Scrub

¾ cup of Himalayan salts

¼ cup of almond oil

¼ cup of sunflower oil

3 drops of rose essential oil

3 drops of neroli essential oil

2 drops of lavender essential oil

Antiaging Bath Bomb

3 tablespoons of citric acid

2 tablespoons of baking soda

2 tablespoons of cornstarch

2 tablespoons of Epsom salts

2 tablespoons of rose powder (pink or red)

1 tablespoon of water

¼ tablespoon of coconut oil

10 drops of neroli essential oil

Skin-Balancing Baths

Skin-Balancing Salt Soak

2 cups of Dead Sea salts
1 cup of Himalayan salts
½ cup of baking soda
1 cup of French green clay
5 drops of geranium essential oil
5 drops of rose essential oil
2 drops of chamomile essential oil

Skin-Balancing Salt Scrub

¾ cup of Himalayan salts
¼ cup of almond oil
¼ cup of sesame seed oil
3 drops of sandalwood essential oil
3 drops of chamomile essential oil

Skin-Balancing Bath Bomb

3 tablespoons of citric acid

2 tablespoons of baking soda

2 tablespoons of cornstarch

2 tablespoons of Epsom salts

2 tablespoons of calendula flower powder

1 tablespoon of water

¼ tablespoon of coconut oil

5 drops of geranium essential oil

5 drops of chamomile essential oil

Cellulite Baths

Cellulite Salt Soak

2 cups of Himalayan salts

1 cup of coarse sea salts

½ cup of baking soda

1 cup of rhassoul clay

5 drops of geranium essential oil

5 drops of grapefruit essential oil

Cellulite Salt Scrub

¾ cup of Dead Sea salts

¼ cup of almond oil

¼ cup of sunflower oil

6 drops of birch (black or yellow) essential oil

Cellulite Bath Bomb

3 tablespoons of citric acid

2 tablespoons of baking soda

2 tablespoons of cornstarch

2 tablespoons of Epsom salts

2 tablespoons of calendula flower powder

1 tablespoon of water

¼ tablespoon of coconut oil

5 drops of geranium essential oil

5 drops of grapefruit essential oil

Cleansing Baths

Cleansing Salt Soak

2 cups of Dead Sea salts

1 cup of Himalayan salts

½ cup of baking soda

1 cup of French green clay

5 drops of chamomile essential oil

5 drops of sandalwood essential oil

Cleansing Salt Scrub

¾ cup of Himalayan salts

¼ cup of almond oil

¼ cup of jojoba oil

3 drops of lemongrass essential oil

3 drops of orange essential oil

Cleansing Bath Bomb

3 tablespoons of citric acid

2 tablespoons of baking soda

2 tablespoons of cornstarch

2 tablespoons of Epsom salts

2 tablespoons of chamomile powder

1 tablespoon of water

¼ tablespoon of coconut oil

10 drops of chamomile essential oil

Detoxifying Salt Soak

1 cup of Dead Sea salts

1 cup of Epsom salts

1 cup of coarse sea salts

½ cup of baking soda

1 cup of French green clay

5 drops of geranium essential oil

5 drops of juniper essential oil

Skin and Beauty

Detoxifying Salt Scrub

¾ cup of Himalayan salts

¼ cup of almond oil

¼ cup of coconut oil

3 drops of lavender essential oil

3 drops of peppermint essential oil

Detoxifying Bath Bomb

3 tablespoons of citric acid

2 tablespoons of baking soda

2 tablespoons of cornstarch

2 tablespoons of Epsom salts

1 tablespoon of water

¼ tablespoon of coconut oil

10 drops of grapefruit essential oil

Baths for Dry Skin

Cracked-Skin Salt Soak 1

2 cups of Dead Sea salts

1 cup of Himalayan salts

½ cup of baking soda

1 cup of French green clay

5 drops of myrrh essential oil

5 drops of lavender essential oil

Cracked-Skin Salt Soak 2

2 cups of Dead Sea salts
1 cup of Epsom salts
½ cup of baking soda
5 drops of benzoin essential oil
5 drops of tea tree essential oil

Dehydrated-Skin Salt Soak

2 cups of Himalayan salts
1 cup of coarse sea salts
½ cup of baking soda
1 cup of rhassoul clay
5 drops of lavender essential oil
5 drops of rose essential oil
2 drops of chamomile essential oil

Dry-Skin Salt Soak

2 cups of Dead Sea salts
1 cup of Himalayan salts
½ cup of baking soda
1 cup of French green clay
10 drops of chamomile essential oil

Dry-Skin Salt Scrub

¾ cup of Himalayan salts

¼ cup of almond oil

¼ cup of sunflower oil

3 drops of rose essential oil

3 drops of neroli essential oil

Dry-Skin Bath Bomb

3 tablespoons of citric acid

2 tablespoons of baking soda

2 tablespoons of cornstarch

2 tablespoons of Epsom salts

1 tablespoon of water

¼ tablespoon of coconut oil

10 drops of jasmine essential oil

Eczema Salt Soak 1

2 cups of Himalayan salts

1 cup of coarse sea salts

½ cup of baking soda

1 cup of fuller's earth clay

5 drops of neroli essential oil

5 drops of lavender essential oil

2 drops of chamomile essential oil

Eczema Salt Soak 2

1 cup of Dead Sea salts

1 cup of Epsom salts

1 cup of coarse sea salts

½ cup of baking soda

1 cup of French green clay

10 drops of juniper essential oil

Eczema Bath Bomb

3 tablespoons of citric acid

2 tablespoons of baking soda

2 tablespoons of cornstarch

2 tablespoons of Epsom salts

2 tablespoons of chamomile flower powder

1 tablespoon of water

¼ tablespoon of coconut oil

5 drops of chamomile essential oil

5 drops of juniper essential oil

Moisturizing Salt Soak

2 cups of Himalayan salts

1 cup of Dead Sea salts

½ cup of baking soda

5 drops of chamomile essential oil

5 drops of rose essential oil

Skin and Beauty

Moisturizing Salt Scrub

¾ cup of Dead Sea salts

¼ cup of avocado oil

¼ cup of olive oil

2 drops of lavender essential oil

2 drops of geranium essential oil

2 drops of cedarwood atlas essential oil

Moisturizing Bath Bomb

3 tablespoons of citric acid

2 tablespoons of baking soda

2 tablespoons of cornstarch

2 tablespoons of Epsom salts

2 tablespoons of rose powder

1 tablespoon of water

¼ tablespoon of coconut oil

5 drops of chamomile essential oil

5 drops of lavender essential oil

Oily Skin Baths

Oily Skin Salt Soak 1

2 cups of Dead Sea salts

1 cup of Himalayan salts

½ cup of baking soda

1 cup of French green clay

5 drops of geranium essential oil

5 drops of sandalwood essential oil

Oily Skin Salt Soak 2

1 cup of Dead Sea salts

1 cup of Epsom salts

1 cup of coarse sea salts

1 cup of French green clay

½ cup of baking soda

5 drops of lavender essential oil

5 drops of sandalwood essential oil

Oily Skin Salt Soak 3

2 cups of Dead Sea salts

1 cup of Epsom salts

½ cup of baking soda

5 drops of bergamot essential oil

5 drops of frankincense essential oil

Skin and Beauty

Oily Skin Salt Scrub 1

¾ cup of Dead Sea salts
¼ cup of almond oil
¼ cup of sunflower oil
3 drops of bergamot essential oil
3 drops of grapefruit essential oil

Oily Skin Salt Scrub 2

¾ cup of Himalayan salts
¼ cup of almond oil
¼ cup of sunflower oil
3 drops of lavender essential oil
3 drops of tea tree essential oil

Oily Skin Bath Bomb

3 tablespoons of citric acid
2 tablespoons of baking soda
2 tablespoons of cornstarch
2 tablespoons of Epsom salts
2 tablespoons of dried lavender
1 tablespoon of water
¼ tablespoon of coconut oil
10 drops of lavender essential oil

Sensitive Skin Baths

Sensitive Skin Salt Soak

2 cups of Himalayan salts

1 cup of coarse sea salts

½ cup of baking soda

5 drops of chamomile essential oil

5 drops of spikenard essential oil

Sensitive Skin Bath Bomb

3 tablespoons of citric acid

2 tablespoons of baking soda

2 tablespoons of cornstarch

2 tablespoons of Epsom salts

1 tablespoon of water

¼ tablespoon of coconut oil

10 drops of rose essential oil

Skin-Smoothing Baths

Skin-Smoothing Salt Soak

2 cups of Himalayan salts
1 cup of coarse sea salts
½ cup of baking soda
1 cup of rhassoul clay
10 drops of neroli essential oil
10 drops of frankincense essential oil

Skin-Smoothing Salt Scrub

¾ cup of Himalayan salts
¼ cup of almond oil
¼ cup of rosehip seed oil
5 drops of neroli essential oil
5 drops of rose essential oil

Skin-Smoothing Bath Bomb

3 tablespoons of citric acid
2 tablespoons of baking soda
2 tablespoons of cornstarch
2 tablespoons of Epsom salts
2 tablespoons of rose powder
1 tablespoon of water
¼ tablespoon of coconut oil
5 drops of carrot seed essential oil
5 drops of frankincense essential oil

CHAPTER 7
MEDITATIVE BATHS

Later in this chapter, I will introduce the concept of setting intentions with healing baths (page 82). A meditative bath is the perfect place for this. While the other sections in this book are more focused on healing specific mental, emotional, or physical ailments, this section is more inspirational and intuitive, with blends designed to take you to a calm state where you can let go of your thoughts and be in the moment.

Practicing meditation every day can make you feel more grounded and happier overall. These meditative baths aren't meant to replace your everyday meditation practice if you have one, but they are a delightful addition to it.

These recipes are a guide for grouping scents in a manner that stimulates your creativity. They might remind you of something you'd like to focus on in your meditation. Either way, this is your chance to be inspired; use your intuition as to which scents speak to you and connect to your intention.

How to Set an Intention for Your Bath

If you're familiar with meditation or yoga, you may already be aware of setting intentions before settling into your meditative state. For those of you who have never done this before, don't fret, it's very easy!

First, draw the bath, toss in the salt soak or bath bomb, dim the lights and light candles, or do whatever it is you need to do to create a peaceful setting for the bath. After everything is set up and you're settled in the tub, start your meditative bath by taking a couple of deep belly breaths. Breathe in through your nose down into your tummy and then breathe out through your nose or mouth. This does two things. First, it relaxes you. Second, breathing in the scents of the essential oils will evoke a certain feeling depending on which ones you are using. While you are doing this, set an intention for the bath in your mind. It could be one word or a phrase. For instance, if I'm feeling anxious for some reason, I may choose for my intention the word "acceptance" or "letting go" to bring me to a calmer state and reduce anxiety. Or, if I'm feeling pretty content, then I may choose "gratefulness" as my intention. You see, how you set your intention is completely up to you, and it could literally be anything. I would just recommend listening to your intuition to see if there's anything that is bothering you, something you may need to let go of, or something you would like to focus on.

Once you state your intention in your mind, focus on it for a deep breath or two, then let it go and clear your mind. Continue to focus on breathing to stay in the present, leaving you in a peaceful and meditative state.

Salt Soaks

When I think of meditative baths, the first thing that comes to mind is a deeply relaxing salt soak with essential oils that set a certain tone or mood.

Patchouli Deep Relaxation Salt Soak

This can be used as a grounding meditation to release anxiety. The combination of patchouli, sweet marjoram, and carrot seed create a deep resonating scent for extreme relaxation and letting go.

1 cup of Dead Sea salts

1 cup of Epsom salts

1 cup of coarse sea salts

½ cup of baking soda

1 cup of French green clay

5 drops of patchouli essential oil

5 drops of sweet marjoram essential oil

2 drops of carrot seed essential oil

Clary Sage Uplifting Salt Soak

Warm and light; deep, yet uplifting. This may seem like an unlikely combination, but somehow it works.

2 cups of Himalayan salts

1 cup of coarse sea salts

½ cup of baking soda

1 cup of rhassoul clay

5 drops of clary sage essential oil

5 drops of lemongrass essential oil

2 drops of benzoin essential oil

Citronella Uplifting Salt Soak

This blend is bright and uplifting, great for inspiration and focusing on creative endeavors.

2 cups of Himalayan salts

1 cup of coarse sea salts

½ cup of baking soda

5 drops of citronella essential oil

5 drops of grapefruit essential oil

2 drops of lemongrass essential oil

Bergamot Grounding Salt Soak

Very grounding, this blend will bring you back down to earth.

2 cups of Himalayan salts
1 cup of coarse sea salts
½ cup of baking soda
1 cup of rhassoul clay
5 drops of bergamot essential oil
5 drops of frankincense essential oil
2 drops of juniper berry essential oil

Rose and Basil Salt Soak

The basil in this blend has the ability to make you more alert, yet the rose brings a dreamy aspect. This is a very positive blend for use earlier in the day or maybe before an event.

2 cups of Dead Sea salts
1 cup of Himalayan salts
½ cup of baking soda
1 cup of French green clay
5 drops of rose essential oil
5 drops of basil essential oil

Geranium and Chamomile Salt Soak

"Comforting" is the word that comes to mind to describe this blend. Let it remind you of home and put you in a happy place.

2 cups of Himalayan salts

1 cup of coarse sea salts

½ cup of baking soda

1 cup of fuller's earth clay

5 drops of geranium essential oil

5 drops of chamomile essential oil

Soothing Frankincense Salt Soak

Deep and soothing, this blend will put you in an extremely meditative state. Perfect right before bedtime.

2 cups of Dead Sea salts

1 cup of Epsom salts

½ cup of baking soda

5 drops of frankincense essential oil

5 drops of lavender essential oil

2 drops of eucalyptus essential oil

Bergamot and Jasmine Salt Soak

This is a very gentle and uplifting blend. Perfect for the morning if you have time to take a bath before work.

1 cup of Dead Sea salts
1 cup of Epsom salts
1 cup of coarse sea salts
½ cup of baking soda
5 drops of bergamot essential oil
5 drops of jasmine essential oil

Cedarwood and Lavender Salt Soak

One of my favorites, this blend evokes the feeling of being taken away at sea over gentle waves—each note of the scents allows you to escape to another place.

2 cups of Himalayan salts
1 cup of coarse sea salts
½ cup of baking soda
1 cup of fuller's earth clay
5 drops of cedarwood atlas essential oil
5 drops of lavender essential oil
2 drops of rose essential oil

Comforting Benzoin Salt Soak

Simple, yet comforting, this blend allows the mind to drift.

2 cups of Dead Sea salts

1 cup of coarse sea salts

½ cup of baking soda

1 cup of rhassoul clay

5 drops of benzoin essential oil

5 drops of patchouli essential oil

Bath Bombs

Bath bombs are another way to enjoy a meditative bath. Just drop one in and soak up the benefits.

Invigorating Bath Bomb

With scents reminiscent of summer, this invigorating blend is best for an early meditation bath.

3 tablespoons of citric acid

2 tablespoons of baking soda

2 tablespoons of cornstarch

2 tablespoons of Epsom salts

1 tablespoon of water

¼ tablespoon of coconut oil

5 drops of marjoram essential oil

5 drops of lemongrass essential oil

Bedtime Bath Bomb

Surround yourself with deep woodsy scents for a late-night bath.

3 tablespoons of citric acid

2 tablespoons of baking soda

2 tablespoons of cornstarch

2 tablespoons of Epsom salts

1 tablespoon of water

¼ tablespoon of coconut oil

5 drops of carrot seed essential oil

5 drops of cedarwood atlas essential oil

Grapefruit and Rose Bath Bomb

This fruity floral blend is inspiring for creative and artistic intentions.

3 tablespoons of citric acid

2 tablespoons of baking soda

2 tablespoons of cornstarch

2 tablespoons of Epsom salts

1 tablespoon of water

¼ tablespoon of coconut oil

5 drops of grapefruit essential oil

5 drops of rose essential oil

Meditative Baths

Stimulating Bath Bomb

The combination of lavender and bergamot is very stimulating. Great for a quick meditative bath before a productive day.

3 tablespoons of citric acid

2 tablespoons of baking soda

2 tablespoons of cornstarch

2 tablespoons of Epsom salts

1 tablespoon of water

¼ tablespoon of coconut oil

5 drops of lavender essential oil

5 drops of bergamot essential oil

Grounding Bath Bomb

Frankincense and patchouli make for a very grounding, earthy combination.

3 tablespoons of citric acid

2 tablespoons of baking soda

2 tablespoons of cornstarch

2 tablespoons of Epsom salts

1 tablespoon of water

¼ tablespoon of coconut oil

5 drops of frankincense essential oil

5 drops of patchouli essential oil

Salt Scrubs

Meditative scrubs...is there such a thing? I think so. Salt scrubs can be extremely relaxing, especially before a bath. Scrub first, then deep meditative relaxation.

Deep Relaxation Salt Scrub

The deep scents of the juniper berry can evoke a deep meditative state.

¾ cup of Dead Sea salts

¼ cup of almond oil

¼ cup of sunflower oil

6 drops of juniper berry essential oil

Comforting Salt Scrub

There's something about the combination of geranium and benzoin together that creates a sense of comfort and peace.

¾ cup of Dead Sea salts

¼ cup of almond oil

¼ cup of sunflower oil

3 drops of geranium essential oil

3 drops of benzoin essential oil

Uplifting Salt Scrub

This is a great scrub to use in the morning to set your mind on the right track for the day.

¾ cup of Dead Sea salts
¼ cup of almond oil
¼ cup of sunflower oil
3 drops of tea tree essential oil
3 drops of lemongrass essential oil

Invigorating Salt Scrub

The mixture of clary sage and peppermint stimulates mental alertness.

¾ cup of Dead Sea salts
¼ cup of almond oil
¼ cup of sunflower oil
3 drops of clary sage essential oil
3 drops of peppermint essential oil

Gentle Salt Scrub

Perfect scrub to put you at ease any time of the day, but especially bedtime.

¾ cup of Dead Sea salts
¼ cup of almond oil
¼ cup of sunflower oil
3 drops of chamomile essential oil
3 drops of rose essential oil

CHAPTER 8
CHAKRAS

The subject of chakras is complex and fascinating. There are seven main chakras in our bodies, each connected to different organs and each aligned along the spine. Every chakra is an energy center representing different areas in our life. The word chakra means "wheel" in Sanskrit, which is basically how the energy moves within each chakra. Since chakras are energy vortexes, when we feel low energy or off it can mean one or more of our chakras are imbalanced. The essential oils associated with the baths below are meant to restore each chakra back to balance. I've also found that setting intentions (page 82) work well here too.

Educating yourself about chakras will help you identify where you may be feeling blocks or imbalances in your life. We're only able to touch on the basics of each chakra in this book, but three books that I highly recommend if you want to learn more are *The Chakra Bible* by Patricia Mercier, *Chakras for Beginners* by David Pond, and *Subtle Aromatherapy* by Patricia Davis.

The Base Chakra

The base chakra is located at the root of the spine and is the color red. It represents our basic necessities such as food, sex, shelter, and security. When your base chakra is unbalanced you may feel physically fatigued or spacey or experience sexual dysfunction from suppression or lust. Other symptoms include overeating and feeling the need to hoard material things such as money. Those with balanced base chakras will feel a deep connection with the earth.

Base Chakra Salt Soak

2 cups of Dead Sea salts

1 cup of Epsom salts

½ cup of baking soda

5 drops of myrrh essential oil

5 drops of patchouli essential oil

Base Chakra Salt Scrub

¾ cup of Himalayan salts

¼ cup of almond oil

¼ cup of sunflower oil

2 drops of myrrh essential oil

2 drops of cedarwood atlas essential oil

2 drops of frankincense essential oil

Base Chakra Bath Bomb

3 tablespoons of citric acid

2 tablespoons of baking soda

2 tablespoons of cornstarch

2 tablespoons of Epsom salts

1 tablespoon of water

¼ tablespoon of coconut oil

10 drops of rosewood essential oil

The Sacral Chakra

The sacral chakra is located at the sacrum and is the color orange. It represents our sexual energy. When your sacral chakra is unbalanced you may feel a lack of sexual energy, anger or fear in romantic relationships, jealousy, and empty sexual encounters. Balanced sacral chakras will feel fulfilled sexual energy, creativity, joy, unconditional love, and deep connections with others.

Sacral Chakra Salt Soak

2 cups of Dead Sea salts

1 cup of Himalayan salts

½ cup of baking soda

1 cup of French green clay

5 drops of jasmine essential oil

5 drops of rose essential oil

Sacral Chakra Salt Scrub

¾ cup of Himalayan salts

¼ cup of almond oil

¼ cup of sunflower oil

2 drops of jasmine essential oil

2 drops of rose essential oil

2 drops of sandalwood essential oil

Sacral Chakra Bath Bomb

3 tablespoons of citric acid

2 tablespoons of baking soda

2 tablespoons of cornstarch

2 tablespoons of Epsom salts

1 tablespoon of water

¼ tablespoon of coconut oil

10 drops of ylang-ylang essential oil

The Solar Plexus Chakra

The solar plexus chakra is located between the navel and sternum, and is the color yellow. It represents our personal identity, power, and self-acceptance. When your solar plexus chakra is out of balance you may experience anger, competitiveness, conflicts, feelings of guilt or shame due to others' expectations, and negative reactions to stress. When balanced, the solar plexus gives us self-assertiveness, discipline, willpower, and the ability to create healthy boundaries and express our individuality.

Solar Plexus Chakra Salt Soak

1 cup of Dead Sea salts
1 cup of Epsom salts
1 cup of coarse sea salts
½ cup of baking soda
5 drops of vetiver essential oil
5 drops of juniper essential oil

Solar Plexus Chakra Salt Scrub

¾ cup of Himalayan salts
¼ cup of almond oil
¼ cup of sunflower oil
3 drops of clary sage essential oil
3 drops of juniper essential oil

Solar Plexus Chakra Bath Bomb

3 tablespoons of citric acid

2 tablespoons of baking soda

2 tablespoons of cornstarch

2 tablespoons of Epsom salts

1 tablespoon of water

¼ tablespoon of coconut oil

10 drops of geranium essential oil

The Heart Chakra

The heart chakra is located in the heart and is the color green. It represents love of nature, creation, and the world around us. When unbalanced you may experience codependency, attachment, insecurity, or suffering in love. When balanced the heart chakra creates unconditional love and acceptance.

Heart Chakra Salt Soak

2 cups of Himalayan salts

1 cup of Dead Sea salts

½ cup of baking soda

1 cup of rhassoul clay

5 drops of rose essential oil

5 drops of neroli essential oil

Heart Chakra Salt Scrub

¾ cup of Himalayan salts

¼ cup of almond oil

¼ cup of sunflower oil

3 drops of melissa essential oil

3 drops of rose essential oil

Heart Chakra Bath Bomb

3 tablespoons of citric acid

2 tablespoons of baking soda

2 tablespoons of cornstarch

2 tablespoons of Epsom salts

1 tablespoon of water

¼ tablespoon of coconut oil

10 drops of jasmine essential oil

The Throat Chakra

The throat chakra is located at the throat and is the color blue. It represents the transition from the physical body to the spiritual realm, as well as our communication with the world. When the throat chakra is unbalanced you may experience difficulties in communicating, defensiveness, anxiety, depression, and the need to seek approval. When balanced, the throat chakra allows you to be authentic and creative in your communication and self-expression.

Throat Chakra Salt Soak

1 cup of Dead Sea salts

1 cup of Epsom salts

1 cup of coarse sea salts

½ cup of baking soda

1 cup of French green clay

10 drops of chamomile essential oil

Throat Chakra Salt Scrub

¾ cup of Himalayan salts

¼ cup of almond oil

¼ cup of sunflower oil

3 drops of lavender essential oil

3 drops of chamomile essential oil

Throat Chakra Bath Bomb

3 tablespoons of citric acid

2 tablespoons of baking soda

2 tablespoons of cornstarch

2 tablespoons of Epsom salts

1 tablespoon of water

¼ tablespoon of coconut oil

10 drops of chamomile essential oil

The Brow Chakra

The brow chakra is located in the forehead and is the color indigo. It represents emotional clarity and intuition. When your brow chakra is out of balance, you may experience headaches, sleep disorders, fear, addiction to drugs and alcohol, and excessive fantasizing. When the brow chakra is balanced it stimulates creative visualization, transcendence, intuition, and the ability to reach higher realms.

Brow Chakra Salt Soak

2 cups of Dead Sea salts

1 cup of Epsom salts

½ cup of baking soda

5 drops of basil essential oil

5 drops of juniper essential oil

Brow Chakra Salt Scrub

¾ cup of Himalayan salts

¼ cup of almond oil

¼ cup of sunflower oil

6 drops of frankincense essential oil

Brow Chakra Bath Bomb

3 tablespoons of citric acid

2 tablespoons of baking soda

2 tablespoons of cornstarch

2 tablespoons of Epsom salts

1 tablespoon of water

¼ tablespoon of coconut oil

10 drops of frankincense essential oil

The Crown Chakra

The crown chakra is located at the top of the head and is the color violet. It represents pure consciousness. When the crown chakra is unbalanced, the ego dominates and directs your life instead of surrendering to the magic of flow. When balanced you experience full awareness, as well as the ability to meditate and surrender to your spirituality.

Crown Chakra Salt Soak

2 cups of Dead Sea salts
1 cup of Epsom salts
½ cup of baking soda
5 drops of rose essential oil
5 drops of jasmine essential oil

Crown Chakra Salt Scrub

¾ cup of Himalayan salts
¼ cup of almond oil
¼ cup of sunflower oil
3 drops of frankincense essential oil
3 drops of ylang-ylang essential oil

Crown Chakra Bath Bomb

3 tablespoons of citric acid

2 tablespoons of baking soda

2 tablespoons of cornstarch

2 tablespoons of Epsom salts

1 tablespoon of water

¼ tablespoon of coconut oil

10 drops of rosewood essential oil

The Aura Chakra

The aura chakra is located above the head and is the color white. This chakra is about reaching true spiritual wisdom and access to your high self.

Aura Chakra Salt Soak

2 cups of Himalayan salts

1 cup of coarse sea salts

½ cup of baking soda

1 cup of fuller's earth clay

10 drops of neroli essential oil

Aura Chakra Salt Scrub

¾ cup of Himalayan salts

¼ cup of almond oil

¼ cup of sunflower oil

6 drops of neroli essential oil

Aura Chakra Bath Bomb

3 tablespoons of citric acid
2 tablespoons of baking soda
2 tablespoons of cornstarch
2 tablespoons of Epsom salts
1 tablespoon of water
¼ tablespoon of coconut oil
10 drops of neroli essential oil

CHAPTER 9
ASTROLOGY

To many people, astrology is nothing more than your monthly horoscope. But it is so much more than that! I recently had my natal chart done and was shocked at not only how accurate it was, but also how it answered questions about myself that I've had all my life. And lo and behold, there are essential oils associated with each sign and planet! Astrology can become pretty complicated, so if you can, I recommend having your natal chart done by an astrologist.

For now we'll just stick with talking about the sun signs, which most everyone is familiar with. You can find your sun sign simply by the date of your birth. Each sign has plants or essential oils that can help restore them back to their true states. There are a few recipes for each sign, based on corresponding personalities and tendencies, as well as positive and negative traits. These recipes are meant to keep each sign balanced.

Aries
(March 21 to April 19)

Aries (the ram) is the feisty, determined go-getter and leader. As innovative pioneers, rams love to start projects and thrive on living in the moment. Because they are very physical and athletic beings, they tend to overexhaust themselves and need to be both restored and soothed.

Aries Soothing Salt Soak

2 cups of Dead Sea salts

1 cup of Epsom salts

½ cup of baking soda

5 drops of rose essential oil

5 drops of geranium essential oil

Aries Restoring Salt Scrub

¾ cup of Dead Sea salts

¼ cup of almond oil

¼ cup of sunflower oil

2 drops of bergamot essential oil

2 drops of orange essential oil

2 drops of ginger essential oil

Aries Balancing Bath Bomb

3 tablespoons of citric acid

2 tablespoons of baking soda

2 tablespoons of cornstarch

2 tablespoons of Epsom salts

1 tablespoon of water

¼ tablespoon of coconut oil

5 drops of geranium essential oil

5 drops of orange essential oil

Taurus
(April 20 to May 20)

Taurus (the bull) loves luxury and the sensual things in life: delicious food, good sex, and owning nice material things. On the other hand, Taurus signs are extremely hard workers. Maybe it's because of this that the bull seems to overindulge in their delights. A little cleanse now and then is key.

Taurus Cleansing Salt Soak

2 cups of Dead Sea salts

1 cup of Epsom salts

½ cup of baking soda

5 drops of lemongrass essential oil

5 drops of fennel essential oil

Taurus Luxurious Salt Scrub

¾ cup of Dead Sea salts

¼ cup of almond oil

¼ cup of sunflower oil

2 drops of rose essential oil

2 drops of jasmine essential oil

2 drops of chamomile essential oil

Taurus Stimulating Bath Bomb

3 tablespoons of citric acid

2 tablespoons of baking soda

2 tablespoons of cornstarch

2 tablespoons of Epsom salts

1 tablespoon of water

¼ tablespoon of coconut oil

5 drops of lemongrass essential oil

5 drops of chamomile essential oil

Gemini
(May 21 to June 20)

Gemini (the twins) is the social intellectual. Gemini love matters of the mind, creating new relationships, and never knowing which journey they'll be on or, for that matter, which side of their personality they'll take with them. Because of their constant need for communication and feeding their mind, anxiety and insomnia can often plague them.

Gemini Calming Salt Soak

2 cups of Dead Sea salts
1 cup of Epsom salts
½ cup of baking soda
5 drops of lavender essential oil
5 drops of benzoin essential oil

Gemini Balancing Salt Scrub

¾ cup of Dead Sea salts
¼ cup of almond oil
¼ cup of sunflower oil
3 drops of basil essential oil
3 drops of peppermint essential oil

Gemini Relaxing Bath Bomb

3 tablespoons of citric acid

2 tablespoons of baking soda

2 tablespoons of cornstarch

2 tablespoons of Epsom salts

1 tablespoon of water

¼ tablespoon of coconut oil

5 drops of lavender essential oil

5 drops of chamomile essential oil

Cancer
(June 22 to July 22)

Cancer (the crab) is a home dweller who loves spending time with family and creating traditions. Crabs can be quite emotional or even moody if under stress, retreating back home where they feel safe. They are very sensitive beings and need to feel that they're protected.

Cancer Serene Salt Soak

2 cups of Dead Sea salts

1 cup of Epsom salts

½ cup of baking soda

5 drops of lavender essential oil

5 drops of sandalwood essential oil

2 drops of jasmine essential oil

Cancer Comforting Salt Scrub

¾ cup of Dead Sea salts

¼ cup of almond oil

¼ cup of sunflower oil

2 drops of benzoin essential oil

2 drops of orange essential oil

2 drops of bergamot essential oil

Cancer Grounding Bath Bomb

3 tablespoons of citric acid

2 tablespoons of baking soda

2 tablespoons of cornstarch

2 tablespoons of Epsom salts

1 tablespoon of water

¼ tablespoon of coconut oil

5 drops of sandalwood essential oil

5 drops of benzoin essential oil

Leo
(July 23 to August 22)

Leo (the lion) is the king. Majestic, athletic, and creative, Leos need to have freedom to follow their pursuits; otherwise, they may suffer from depression. The sun, heart, and warmth play a big role in their lives, so outdoor activity followed by a cool rinse and relaxation are very important.

Leo Warming Salt Soak

2 cups of Dead Sea salts
1 cup of Epsom salts
½ cup of baking soda
5 drops of benzoin essential oil
5 drops of chamomile essential oil
2 drops of orange essential oil

Leo Cooling Salt Scrub

¾ cup of Dead Sea salts
¼ cup of almond oil
¼ cup of sunflower oil
2 drops of eucalyptus essential oil
2 drops of citronella essential oil
2 drops of bergamot essential oil

Leo Uplifting Bath Bomb

3 tablespoons of citric acid
2 tablespoons of baking soda
2 tablespoons of cornstarch
2 tablespoons of Epsom salts
1 tablespoon of water
¼ tablespoon of coconut oil
5 drops of chamomile essential oil
5 drops of bergamot essential oil
2 drops of orange essential oil

Virgo
(August 23 to September 21)

Virgo (the virgin) is the healer of the zodiac. Born to serve others, Virgos are earthy perfectionists. Health is very important to them, to the point that they can either develop hypochondriac tendencies or go to the other extreme by putting their own health aside to serve others.

Virgo Nurturing Salt Soak

2 cups of Dead Sea salts
1 cup of Epsom salts
½ cup of baking soda
5 drops of lavender essential oil
5 drops of carrot seed essential oil
2 drops of chamomile essential oil

Virgo Indulgence Salt Scrub

¾ cup of Dead Sea salts

¼ cup of almond oil

¼ cup of sunflower oil

3 drops of rose essential oil

3 drops of jasmine essential oil

Virgo Healing Bath Bomb

3 tablespoons of citric acid

2 tablespoons of baking soda

2 tablespoons of cornstarch

2 tablespoons of Epsom salts

1 tablespoon of water

¼ tablespoon of coconut oil

5 drops of rose essential oil

5 drops of lavender essential oil

Libra
(September 22 to October 23)

Libra (the scales) is a lover of ideals, beauty, and companionship. Libras are charming and aim to appear the best almost to the point of coming off vain. Good taste and refinement are very important to Libras, although indulging in the luxuries of life can throw them off balance.

Libra Rebalancing Salt Soak

2 cups of Dead Sea salts

1 cup of Epsom salts

½ cup of baking soda

5 drops of rosemary essential oil

5 drops of bergamot essential oil

2 drops of citronella essential oil

Libra Beautifying Salt Scrub

¾ cup of Dead Sea salts

¼ cup of almond oil

¼ cup of sunflower oil

2 drops of rose essential oil

2 drops of carrot seed essential oil

2 drops of ylang-ylang essential oil

Libra Luxurious Bath Bomb

3 tablespoons of citric acid
2 tablespoons of baking soda
2 tablespoons of cornstarch
2 tablespoons of Epsom salts
1 tablespoon of water
¼ tablespoon of coconut oil
5 drops of ylang-ylang essential oil
5 drops of jasmine essential oil

Scorpio
(October 24 to November 21)

Scorpio (the scorpion) is the intuitive investigator, always probing into the secretive, mysterious sides to life. Stubborn, loyal, and emotional, Scorpios can sometimes let their feelings get the best of them.

Scorpio Deep Relaxation Salt Soak

2 cups of Dead Sea salts
1 cup of Epsom salts
½ cup of baking soda
5 drops of patchouli essential oil
5 drops of sandalwood essential oil
2 drops of grapefruit essential oil

Astrology

Scorpio Intoxicating Salt Scrub

¾ cup of Dead Sea salts

¼ cup of almond oil

¼ cup of sunflower oil

2 drops of bergamot essential oil

2 drops of benzoin seed essential oil

2 drops of jasmine essential oil

Scorpio Aphrodisiac Bath Bomb

3 tablespoons of citric acid

2 tablespoons of baking soda

2 tablespoons of cornstarch

2 tablespoons of Epsom salts

1 tablespoon of water

¼ tablespoon of coconut oil

5 drops of ylang-ylang essential oil

5 drops of jasmine essential oil

Sagittarius
(November 22 to December 21)

Sagittarius (the archer) is the free-spirited intellectual searching for the truth of the matter. Charming and optimistic, Sags can become depressed when they feel repressed or trapped. Conversely they have a tendency to push them themselves too far on their explorations, leaving them exhausted.

Sagittarius Replenishing Salt Soak

2 cups of Dead Sea salts

1 cup of Epsom salts

½ cup of baking soda

5 drops of lavender essential oil

5 drops of rose essential oil

Sagittarius Invigorating Salt Scrub

¾ cup of Dead Sea salts

¼ cup of almond oil

¼ cup of sunflower oil

2 drops of black pepper essential oil

2 drops of clary sage essential oil

2 drops of marjoram essential oil

Sagittarius Calming Bath Bomb

3 tablespoons of citric acid

2 tablespoons of baking soda

2 tablespoons of cornstarch

2 tablespoons of Epsom salts

1 tablespoon of water

¼ tablespoon of coconut oil

5 drops of ylang-ylang essential oil

5 drops of lavender essential oil

2 drops of chamomile essential oil

Capricorn
(December 22 to January 19)

Capricorn (the goat) is determined, pragmatic, and always has an eye on the goal and the accompanying rewards that come with it. Being hardworking and loyal, with the need to feel useful can often leave them feeling depleted and drained. Self-pampering is needed for Caps every once in a while to stay balanced.

Capricorn Pampering Salt Soak

2 cups of Dead Sea salts

1 cup of Epsom salts

½ cup of baking soda

5 drops of benzoin essential oil

5 drops of rose essential oil

2 drops of jasmine essential oil

Capricorn Reviving Salt Scrub

¾ cup of Dead Sea salts

¼ cup of almond oil

¼ cup of sunflower oil

2 drops of lemongrass pepper essential oil

2 drops of bergamot essential oil

2 drops of orange essential oil

Capricorn Balancing Bath Bomb

3 tablespoons of citric acid

2 tablespoons of baking soda

2 tablespoons of cornstarch

2 tablespoons of Epsom salts

1 tablespoon of water

¼ tablespoon of coconut oil

5 drops of benzoin essential oil

5 drops of orange essential oil

Aquarius
(January 20 to February 18)

The Aquarius (the water bearer) is the eccentric, forward-thinking humanitarian of the zodiac. Water bearers are offbeat, individualistic, and sometimes unpredictable. Aloof and nonconformist, at extremes Aquarians can sometimes turn negative and reclusive when things don't go their way.

Aquarius Meditating Salt Soak

2 cups of Dead Sea salts

1 cup of Epsom salts

½ cup of baking soda

5 drops of neroli essential oil

5 drops of rose essential oil

2 drops of lavender essential oil

Aquarius Grounding Salt Scrub

¾ cup of Dead Sea salts

¼ cup of almond oil

¼ cup of sunflower oil

2 drops of sandalwood essential oil

2 drops of oakmoss essential oil

2 drops of benzoin essential oil

Aquarius Uplifting Bath Bomb

3 tablespoons of citric acid

2 tablespoons of baking soda

2 tablespoons of cornstarch

2 tablespoons of Epsom salts

1 tablespoon of water

¼ tablespoon of coconut oil

5 drops of rose essential oil

5 drops of bergamot essential oil

Pisces
(February 19 to March 20)

Pisces (the fish) are dreamy, creative, and deeply emotional souls. They are artistic and intuitive, relying more on their feelings than other signs. Sensitive, they can sometimes stay in their fantasy world instead of dealing with reality. They also are big givers and lovers, yet because of this they have a tendency to be self-sacrificing.

Pisces Centering Salt Soak

2 cups of Dead Sea salts

1 cup of Epsom salts

½ cup of baking soda

5 drops of melissa essential oil

5 drops of rose essential oil

2 drops of geranium essential oil

Pisces Therapeutic Salt Scrub

¾ cup of Dead Sea salts

¼ cup of almond oil

¼ cup of sunflower oil

2 drops of chamomile essential oil

2 drops of rose essential oil

2 drops of grapefruit essential oil

Pisces Dreamy Bath Bomb

3 tablespoons of citric acid

2 tablespoons of baking soda

2 tablespoons of cornstarch

2 tablespoons of Epsom salts

1 tablespoon of water

¼ tablespoon of coconut oil

5 drops of jasmine essential oil

5 drops of melissa essential oil

CHAPTER 10
APHRODISIAC BATHS

I couldn't write a book about bath salt soaks without including a section on aphrodisiac soaks. Sex, whether we like it or not, plays a huge role in our lives. Sadly, there are so many negative connotations to sex. Growing up, many of us we're taught that sex is essentially bad by focusing on all the negative consequences that can come from it. And while those consequences may be true, sex can also be a very beautiful experience. Mother earth can enhance that experience...with aphrodisiac scents. It doesn't matter where you are in your life. Whether you're in a relationship or not, these particular soaks are about allowing you to be you and to feel good about who you are.

Rose

Rose might be the scent most often associated with love and sex. The scent of the heart chakra, it appeals to both women and men and seems to get people in the mood. It is a very gentle scent, evoking feelings of acceptance and love rather than lust.

Rose Salt Soak

1 cup of dried rose petals

2 cups of Dead Sea salts

2 cups of Himalayan salts

½ cup of baking soda

1 cup of French green clay

10 drops of rose essential oil

Jasmine

Jasmine is rose's exotic sister scent. They are both very feminine, but jasmine always conjures feelings of the East. I love the smell of jasmine. It's considered the ultimate aphrodisiac oil, along with rose. Very delicate, it puts one at ease, almost like a good glass of wine.

Delicate Jasmine Salt Soak

½ cup of dried jasmine flowers

2 cups of Himalayan salts

1 cup of coarse sea salts

½ cup of baking soda

1 cup of rhassoul clay

10 drops of jasmine essential oil

Patchouli

Patchouli gets a bad rap. Ask around and you'll find that most people in the Gen X and millennial generations associate patchouli as a pungent oil that Dad used to wear back in the '60s and '70s. Or that it's only for hippies. I take offense to that! Yes, it was a popular oil among hippies and yes, it has a very strong scent, but if people took away their preconceived notions regarding patchouli, they would be surprised at how much they enjoyed it. It has a dark, earthy sexuality to it. It may appeal more to men, but women can enjoy it too.

Patchouli Salt Soak

2 cups of Dead Sea salts

1 cup of coarse sea salts

½ cup of baking soda

10 drops of patchouli essential oil

Bergamot

Bergamot isn't one of the more popular aphrodisiac oils, but it should be. It's a very romantic oil, reminiscent of Rome, an ancient city that is all about romance, the senses, and, on an understated level, sex. It evokes the charming, romantic side of sex—dating, candlelit dinners, and getting to know someone.

Bergamot Salt Soak

1 cup of Dead Sea salts
1 cup of Epsom salts
1 cup of coarse sea salts
½ cup of baking soda
10 drops of bergamot essential oil

CHAPTER 11
BATH RECIPES FOR PREGNANCY

Baths are a gentle way for pregnant women to give their bodies a well-deserved break and take time to themselves before the baby comes. As I stated earlier in the book, it's important for pregnant women to be extremely careful with essential oils, as some can be downright dangerous. For that reason, I've included a few recipes that are safe for them to use. By no means are these the only essential oils available to pregnant women, but they are the ones that are considered safe. If you are pregnant and want to learn more about other essential oils, I recommend booking an appointment with an aromatherapist so they can cater specific oils to your specific needs.

These recipes are safe for pregnant women to use any time throughout their pregnancy.

Neroli and Mandarin Pregnancy Salt Soak

2 cups of Himalayan salts

1 cup of coarse sea salts

½ cup of baking soda

3 drops of neroli essential oil

3 drops of mandarin essential oil

Neroli and Mandarin Pregnancy Salt Scrub

¾ cup of Dead Sea salts

¼ cup of almond oil

¼ cup of sunflower oil

3 drops of neroli essential oil

3 drops of mandarin essential oil

Neroli and Mandarin Pregnancy Bath Bomb

2 tablespoons of baking soda

2 tablespoons of cornstarch

2 tablespoons of Epsom salts

1 tablespoon of water

¼ tablespoon of coconut oil

3 drops of neroli essential oil

3 drops of mandarin essential oil

These recipes are safe for pregnant women to use after four to five months of pregnancy.

Rose and Chamomile Pregnancy Salt Soak

2 cups of Himalayan salts

1 cup of coarse sea salts

½ cup of baking soda

5 drops of rose essential oil

5 drops of Roman chamomile essential oil

Rose and Chamomile Pregnancy Salt Scrub

¾ cup of Dead Sea salts

¼ cup of almond oil

¼ cup of sunflower oil

3 drops of rose essential oil

3 drops of chamomile essential oil

Rose and Chamomile Pregnancy Bath Bomb

2 tablespoons of baking soda

2 tablespoons of cornstarch

2 tablespoons of Epsom salts

1 tablespoon of water

¼ tablespoon of coconut oil

3 drops of rose essential oil

3 drops of chamomile essential oil

Lavender Pregnancy Salt Soak

2 cups of Himalayan salts

1 cup of coarse sea salts

½ cup of baking soda

6 drops of lavender essential oil

Lavender Pregnancy Salt Scrub

¾ cup of Dead Sea salts

¼ cup of almond oil

¼ cup of sunflower oil

3 drops of lavender essential oil

Lavender Pregnancy Bath Bomb

2 tablespoons of baking soda
2 tablespoons of cornstarch
2 tablespoons of Epsom salts
1 tablespoon of water
¼ tablespoon of coconut oil
3 drops of lavender essential oil

CHAPTER 12
BATH BLENDS FOR HIM

Men need pampering too. Some may not like to admit it, but deep down they can't resist a relaxing bath, especially if it's filled with scents that are outdoorsy and grounding. So if you're a man, this section is especially for you. And ladies, if you think the men in your life might benefit from much-needed relaxation, these recipe make great gifts.

Salt Soaks

Perfect for easing sore muscles after a long day of work or an intense workout.

Clary Sage and Lavender Salt Soak

1 cup of Dead Sea salts
1 cup of Epsom salts
1 cup of coarse sea salts
½ cup of baking soda
5 drops of clary sage essential oil
5 drops of lavender essential oil
2 drops of rosemary essential oil

Cedarwood and Bergamot Salt Soak

1 cup of Dead Sea salts
1 cup of Epsom salts
1 cup of coarse sea salts
½ cup of baking soda
5 drops of cedarwood atlas essential oil
5 drops of bergamot essential oil
2 drops of rosemary essential oil

Frankincense and Benzoin Salt Soak

1 cup of Dead Sea salts

1 cup of Epsom salts

1 cup of coarse sea salts

½ cup of baking soda

5 drops of frankincense essential oil

5 drops of benzoin essential oil

Patchouli and Oakmoss Salt Soak

1 cup of Dead Sea salts

1 cup of Epsom salts

1 cup of coarse sea salts

½ cup of baking soda

5 drops of patchouli atlas essential oil

5 drops of oakmoss essential oil

Salt Scrubs

These salt scrubs are all on the more invigorating side with masculine scents like tea tree, clary sage, and bergamot.

Tea Tree Salt Scrub

¾ cup of Dead Sea salts

¼ cup of almond oil

¼ cup of sunflower oil

6 drops of tea tree essential oil

Clary Sage Salt Scrub

¾ cup of Dead Sea salts

¼ cup of almond oil

¼ cup of sunflower oil

6 drops of clary sage essential oil

Bergamot Salt Scrub

¾ cup of Dead Sea salts

¼ cup of almond oil

¼ cup of sunflower oil

6 drops of bergamot essential oil

Bath Bombs

Since most men seem to love science experiments or anything that involves explosions, these bath bombs may be the best way to entice your man into taking a bath.

Rosemary Bath Bomb

3 tablespoons of citric acid

2 tablespoons of baking soda

2 tablespoons of cornstarch

2 tablespoons of Epsom salts

½ tablespoon of dried rosemary

1 tablespoon of water

¼ tablespoon of coconut oil

10 drops of rosemary essential oil

Peppermint Bath Bomb

4 tablespoons of citric acid
2 tablespoons of baking soda
2 tablespoons of cornstarch
2 tablespoons of Epsom salts
2 tablespoons of dried alfalfa powder (for green color)
1 tablespoon of water
¼ tablespoon of coconut oil
10 drops of peppermint essential oil

Cedarwood Bath Bomb

4 tablespoons of citric acid
2 tablespoons of baking soda
2 tablespoons of cornstarch
2 tablespoons of Epsom salts
1 tablespoon of water
¼ tablespoon of coconut oil
10 drops of cedarwood atlas essential oil

CHAPTER 13
SEASONAL BATHS

Just as the seasons change, so do our needs for comfort and wellness. Baths can be added to your wellness routine as a preventative measure against typical seasonal ailments such as the flu, allergies, and even sunburns. Or, a relaxing bath can be the perfect way to take advantage of the scents and serenities each season has to offer.

Winter

The cold months make for the most rewarding bath season. Who doesn't want to soak in a hot tub while it's freezing outside? Winter salt soaks are also beneficial as a remedy for flu and cold season. In the Ailments chapter (page 26), we covered various baths that protect against viral infections that are typical this time of year.

Here are some additional soaks to help prevent a cold or flu from progressing. Intoxicating scents like eucalyptus and peppermint have a warming quality.

Combining these baths with exercise and good nutrition should keep you in good health and able to bypass the normal illnesses that seem to run rampant during the winter. Make sure to get plenty of sleep after bathing and, most importantly, stay warm.

Winter Flu Prevention Salt Soak

1 cup of Dead Sea salts
1 cup of Epsom salts
1 cup of coarse sea salts
½ cup of baking soda
5 drops of eucalyptus essential oil
5 drops of peppermint essential oil
2 drops of rosemary essential oil

Winter Flu Prevention Bath Bomb

3 tablespoons of citric acid
2 tablespoons of baking soda
2 tablespoons of cornstarch
2 tablespoons of Epsom salts
1 tablespoon of water
¼ tablespoon of coconut oil
5 drops of eucalyptus essential oil
5 drops of peppermint essential oil
2 drops of rosemary essential oil

Warming Winter Salt Soak

1 cup of Dead Sea salts
1 cup of Epsom salts
1 cup of coarse sea salts
½ cup of baking soda
1 cup of French green clay
5 drops of benzoin essential oil
5 drops of cedarwood atlas essential oil
2 drops of lavender essential oil

Warming Winter Salt Scrub

¾ cup of Dead Sea salts
¼ cup of almond oil
¼ drops of benzoin essential oil
3 drops of cedarwood atlas essential oil
3 drops of lavender essential oil

Warming Winter Bath Bomb

2 tablespoons of baking soda
2 tablespoons of cornstarch
2 tablespoons of Epsom salts
1 tablespoon of water
¼ tablespoon of coconut oil
5 drops of benzoin essential oil
5 drops of cedarwood atlas essential oil
2 drops of lavender essential oil

Uplifting Winter Salt Soak

2 cups of Himalayan salts

1 cup of coarse sea salts

½ cup of baking soda

5 drops of bergamot essential oil

5 drops of orange essential oil

Uplifting Winter Salt Scrub

¾ cup of Dead Sea salts

½ cup of safflower oil

3 drops of bergamot essential oil

3 drops of orange essential oil

Uplifting Winter Bath Bomb

3 tablespoons of citric acid

2 tablespoons of baking soda

2 tablespoons of cornstarch

2 tablespoons of Epsom salts

2 tablespoons of chamomile flower powder (for yellow color)

1 tablespoon of water

¼ tablespoon of coconut oil

5 drops of bergamot essential oil

5 drops of orange essential oil

Spring

Spring baths are filled with rejuvenating floral scents of rose and jasmine and chamomile. Check the Floral Baths chapter (page 154), for additional quintessential spring soaks. Spring is also the time for allergies. In many instances, allergies (or any ailment, for that matter) can be brought on by stress. Relaxing in a bath is ideal for reducing a stress-induced allergy flare-up. Chamomile is also beneficial for combating hay fever. You'll find a chamomile blend here, and more allergy-prevention soaks in the Ailments chapter (page 26). Also, if you do have a major bout of allergies, stay clear of anything with artificial fragrances, including perfume and candles. I had a horrible allergy season years ago and it was due to being exposed to an array of candles that were burning daily in a store I worked in.

Brighter Days Salt Soak

2 cups of Himalayan salts
1 cup of coarse sea salts
½ cup of baking soda
1 cup of rhassoul clay
5 drops of geranium essential oil
5 drops of lemongrass essential oil

Brighter Days Salt Scrub

¾ cup of Himalayan salts
½ cup of sunflower oil
3 drops of geranium essential oil
3 drops of lemongrass essential oil

Brighter Days Bath Bomb

3 tablespoons of citric acid

2 tablespoons of baking soda

2 tablespoons of cornstarch

2 tablespoons of Epsom salts

1 tablespoon of water

¼ tablespoon of coconut oil

5 drops of geranium essential oil

5 drops of lemongrass essential oil

Exotic Spring Salt Soak

2 cups of Himalayan salts

1 cup of coarse sea salts

½ cup of baking soda

1 cup of fuller's earth clay

5 drops of juniper berry essential oil

5 drops of jasmine essential oil

Exotic Spring Salt Scrub

¾ cup of Himalayan salts

¼ cup of almond oil

¼ cup of safflower oil

4 drops of jasmine essential oil

2 drops of juniper berry essential oil

Exotic Spring Bath Bomb

3 tablespoons of citric acid

2 tablespoons of baking soda

2 tablespoons of cornstarch

2 tablespoons of Epsom salts

1 tablespoon of water

¼ tablespoon of coconut oil

5 drops of jasmine essential oil

5 drops of juniper essential oil

Rejuvenating Spring Salt Soak

2 cups of Dead Sea salts

2 cups of Himalayan salts

½ cup of baking soda

1 cup of French green clay

5 drops of chamomile essential oil

5 drops of rose essential oil

2 drops of orange essential oil

Rejuvenating Spring Salt Scrub

¾ cup of Dead Sea salts

¼ cup of almond oil

¼ cup of safflower oil

2 drops of chamomile essential oil

2 drops of rose essential oil

2 drops of orange essential oil

Rejuvenating Spring Bath Bomb

3 tablespoons of citric acid

2 tablespoons of baking soda

2 tablespoons of cornstarch

2 tablespoons of Epsom salts

1 tablespoon of water

¼ tablespoon of coconut oil

5 drops of chamomile essential oil

5 drops of rose essential oil

2 drops of orange essential oil

Summer

Summer is my favorite time of year. I love the sun. I love going to the beach. I love being warm. While a hot bath isn't exactly on my mind in the summer, a nice lukewarm bath with summer scents is always a pleasant way to end the day. And if you do happen to get a little too much sun, a cool to lukewarm bath with healing salts and oils will soothe your skin.

Cooling Summer Salt Soak (for Sun-Exposed Skin)

2 cups of Himalayan salts

1 cup of coarse sea salts

½ cup of baking soda

½ cup of dried calendula flowers

5 drops of carrot seed essential oil

5 drops of calendula essential oil

Cooling Summer Bath Bomb

3 tablespoons of citric acid

2 tablespoons of baking soda

2 tablespoons of cornstarch

2 tablespoons of Epsom salts

½ cup of dried calendula flowers

1 tablespoon of water

¼ tablespoon of coconut oil

5 drops of calendula essential oil

5 drops of carrot seed essential oil

Summer Holiday Salt Soak

2 cups of Himalayan salts

1 cup of coarse sea salts

½ cup of baking soda

5 drops of grapefruit essential oil

5 drops of citronella essential oil

2 drops of lemongrass essential oil

Summer Holiday Salt Scrub

¾ cup of Himalayan salts

¼ cup of almond oil

¼ drops of grapefruit essential oil

3 drops of citronella essential oil

3 drops of lemongrass essential oil

Summer Holiday Bath Bomb

3 tablespoons of citric acid

2 tablespoons of baking soda

2 tablespoons of cornstarch

2 tablespoons of Epsom salts

1 tablespoon of water

¼ tablespoon of coconut oil

5 drops of grapefruit essential oil

5 drops of citronella essential oil

2 drops of lemongrass essential oil

Beach Salt Soak

2 cups of Dead Sea salts

1 cup of coarse sea salts

½ cup of baking soda

5 drops of geranium essential oil

5 drops of cedarwood atlas essential oil

2 drops of juniper berry essential oil

Beach Salt Scrub

¾ cup of Dead Sea salts

½ cup of safflower oil

2 drops of geranium essential oil

2 drops of cedarwood atlas essential oil

2 drops of juniper berry essential oil

Beach Bath Bomb

3 tablespoons of citric acid

2 tablespoons of baking soda

2 tablespoons of cornstarch

2 tablespoons of Epsom salts

1 tablespoon of water

¼ tablespoon of coconut oil

5 drops of geranium essential oil

5 drops of cedarwood atlas essential oil

2 drops of juniper berry essential oil

Fall

Toward the end of summer, I think most of us lust after crisp fall days, a break from the heat, and a transition into the holiday season. What comes to mind when I think of fall? Hot tea, warm blankets, soft sweaters, and warm spicy scents reminiscent of November and early December.

Fall Comfort Salt Soak

1 cup of Dead Sea salts

1 cup of Epsom salts

1 cup of coarse sea salts

½ cup of baking soda

1 cup of French green clay

5 drops of patchouli essential oil

5 drops of rose essential oil

2 drops of lavender essential oil

Fall Comfort Salt Scrub

¾ cup of Dead Sea salts

½ cup of almond oil

2 drops of patchouli essential oil

2 drops of rose essential oil

2 drops of lavender berry essential oil

Fall Comfort Bath Bomb

3 tablespoons of citric acid

2 tablespoons of baking soda

2 tablespoons of cornstarch

2 tablespoons of Epsom salts

1 tablespoon of water

¼ tablespoon of coconut oil

5 drops of patchouli essential oil

5 drops of rose essential oil

2 drops of lavender essential oil

Woodsy Fall Salt Soak

2 cups of Dead Sea salts

1 cup of Epsom salts

½ cup of baking soda

5 drops of sandalwood essential oil

5 drops of oakmoss essential oil

2 drops of cedarwood atlas essential oil

Woodsy Fall Salt Scrub

¾ cup of Dead Sea salts

½ cup of almond oil

2 drops of sandalwood essential oil

2 drops of oakmoss essential oil

2 drops of cedarwood atlas essential oil

Woodsy Fall Bath Bomb

3 tablespoons of citric acid

2 tablespoons of baking soda

2 tablespoons of cornstarch

2 tablespoons of Epsom salts

1 tablespoon of water

¼ tablespoon of coconut oil

5 drops of sandalwood essential oil

5 drops of oakmoss essential oil

2 drops of cedarwood atlas essential oil

Spicy Fall Salt Soak

1 cup of Dead Sea salts

1 cup of Epsom salts

1 cup of coarse sea salts

½ cup of baking soda

1 cup of French green clay

5 drops of benzoin essential oil

5 drops of orange essential oil

2 drops of cinnamon essential oil

Spicy Fall Salt Scrub

¾ cup of Dead Sea salts

½ cup of almond oil

2 drops of benzoin essential oil

2 drops of orange essential oil

2 drops of cinnamon essential oil

Spicy Fall Bath Bomb

3 tablespoons of citric acid

2 tablespoons of baking soda

2 tablespoons of cornstarch

2 tablespoons of Epsom salts

1 tablespoon of water

¼ tablespoon of coconut oil

5 drops of benzoin essential oil

5 drops of orange essential oil

2 drops of cinnamon essential oil

CHAPTER 14
FLORAL BATHS

Spring and summer are the best times to utilize floral baths as the floral energies are more aligned with these two seasons. Of course, feel free to do them any time of year. An intoxicating rose or jasmine bath could be a great way to combat the dreariness of winter.

Salt Soaks

These floral salt soaks are the ultimate luxury with actual flowers and petals added. They make lovely gifts, party favors, or wedding favors as well, when divided into small decorative muslin bags.

Note: Because there are a good amount of flowers in these soaks, it's advisable to put a portion of the soak in a small muslin bag and then drop it into the bath. This way, the flowers don't get stuck in the drain and in the tub.

Rose Salt Soak

2 cups of Dead Sea salts

2 cups of Himalayan salts

½ cup of baking soda

1 cup of dried rose petals

1 cup of French green clay

10 drops of rose essential oil

Chamomile Salt Soak

2 cups of Himalayan salts

1 cup of coarse sea salts

½ cup of baking soda

1 cup of dried chamomile petals

1 cup of fuller's earth clay

10 drops of chamomile essential oil

Lavender Salt Soak

2 cups of Himalayan salts

1 cup of coarse sea salts

½ cup of baking soda

1 cup of dried lavender petals

1 cup of rhassoul clay

10 drops of lavender essential oil

Calendula Salt Soak

2 cups of Dead Sea salts

1 cup of Epsom salts

½ cup of baking soda

1 cup of dried calendula petals

10 drops of calendula essential oil

Jasmine Salt Soak

2 cups of Himalayan salts

1 cup of coarse sea salts

½ cup of baking soda

1 cup of dried jasmine petals

10 drops of jasmine essential oil

Delicate Floral Blend Salt Soak

2 cups of Dead Sea salts

2 cups of Himalayan salts

½ cup of baking soda

½ cup of dried jasmine petals

½ cup of dried rose petals

1 cup of French green clay

5 drops of jasmine essential oil

5 drops of rose essential oil

Calming Floral Blend

2 cups of Himalayan salts

1 cup of coarse sea salts

½ cup of baking soda

½ cup of dried calendula petals

½ cup of dried chamomile petals

5 drops of calendula essential oil

5 drops of chamomile essential oil

Salt Scrubs

These floral salt scrubs will make your day and bring a smile to your face. I honestly can't think of anything more luxurious than treating yourself to the Rose Restoring Salt Scrub and then topping it off with the Delicate Floral Blend Salt Soak. Plus, the carrier oils in these scrubs are very lightly scented, letting the scents of the floral essential oils shine.

Delicate Floral Salt Scrub

¾ cup of Dead Sea salts

¼ cup of safflower oil

¼ cup of sunflower oil

3 drops of rose essential oil

3 drops of jasmine essential oil

Lavender Relaxation Salt Scrub

¾ cup of Dead Sea salts

¼ cup of almond oil

¼ cup of sunflower oil

6 drops of lavender essential oil

Gentle Calendula Salt Scrub

¾ cup of Himalayan salts

¼ cup of almond oil

¼ cup of jojoba nut oil

6 drops of calendula essential oil

Simple Calming Chamomile Salt Scrub

¾ cup of Dead Sea salts

½ cup of safflower oil

6 drops of chamomile essential oil

Rose Restoring Salt Scrub

¾ cup of Himalayan salts

¼ cup of almond oil

¼ cup of rosehip oil

6 drops of rose essential oil

Calming Floral Salt Scrub

¾ cup of Dead Sea salts

¼ cup of almond oil

¼ cup of sunflower oil

3 drops of chamomile essential oil

3 drops of calendula essential oil

Bath Bombs

These bath bombs use minimal amounts of flowers and make adorable gifts. If you're concerned about cleanup, consider leaving the flowers out (the flower powder will be fine). However, with the small amount used in each recipe, it shouldn't be an issue.

Jasmine

3 tablespoons of citric acid

2 tablespoons of Epsom salts

2 tablespoons of baking soda

2 tablespoons of cornstarch

2 tablespoons of dried jasmine flowers

1 tablespoon of water

¼ tablespoon of coconut oil

10 drops of jasmine essential oil

Rose

4 tablespoons of citric acid
2 tablespoons of Epsom salts
2 tablespoons of baking soda
2 tablespoons of cornstarch
1 tablespoon of dried rose petals
2 tablespoons of dried rose powder
1 tablespoon of water
¼ tablespoon of coconut oil
10 drops of rose essential oil

Chamomile

4 tablespoons of citric acid
2 tablespoons of Epsom salts
2 tablespoons of baking soda
2 tablespoons of cornstarch
1 tablespoon of dried chamomile petals
2 tablespoons of dried chamomile powder
1 tablespoon of water
¼ tablespoon of coconut oil
10 drops of chamomile essential oil

Lavender

4 tablespoons of citric acid

2 tablespoons of Epsom salts

2 tablespoons of baking soda

2 tablespoons of cornstarch

1 tablespoon of dried lavender petals

2 tablespoons of dried lavender powder

1 tablespoon of water

¼ tablespoon of coconut oil

10 drops of lavender essential oil

Calendula

4 tablespoons of citric acid

2 tablespoons of Epsom salts

2 tablespoons of baking soda

2 tablespoons of cornstarch

1 tablespoon of dried calendula petals

2 tablespoons of dried calendula powder

1 tablespoon of water

¼ tablespoon of coconut oil

10 drops of calendula essential oil

Delicate Floral Bath Bomb

4 tablespoons of citric acid

2 tablespoons of Epsom salts

2 tablespoons of baking soda

2 tablespoons of cornstarch

1 tablespoon of dried jasmine petals

2 tablespoons of dried rose powder

1 tablespoon of water

¼ tablespoon of coconut oil

5 drops of jasmine essential oil

5 drops of rose essential oil

Calming Floral Bath Bomb

4 tablespoons of citric acid

2 tablespoons of Epsom salts

2 tablespoons of baking soda

2 tablespoons of cornstarch

1 tablespoon of dried calendula petals

2 tablespoons of dried chamomile powder

1 tablespoon of water

¼ tablespoon of coconut oil

5 drops of calendula essential oil

5 drops of calendula essential oil

CHAPTER 15
BATHS FROM AROUND THE WORLD

I've always been fascinated by ancient cultures and how they used natural elements for health and beauty. Now natural beauty is making a comeback, and much of it has been derived from cultures of the past.

There's also something very enticing about scents that evoke a sense of place. Isn't it amazing how you can travel across the world, and when you smell the scent of that destination at home, it brings you suddenly back?

The following bath salt recipes evoke time and place for a sensual bath that transports you from daily cares.

Ancient Egyptian Salt Soak

2 cups of Dead Sea salts

1 cup of coarse sea salts

½ cup of baking soda

1 cup of rhassoul clay

5 drops of frankincense essential oil

5 drops of myrrh essential oil

2 drops of lavender essential oil

Ancient Roman Salt Soak

2 cups of Dead Sea salts

1 cup of Epsom salts

½ cup of baking soda

5 drops of frankincense essential oil

5 drops of myrrh essential oil

Modern Roman Salt Soak

2 cups of Dead Sea salts

1 cup of Epsom salts

½ cup of baking soda

5 drops of bergamot essential oil

5 drops of sage essential oil

French Salt Soak

2 cups of Dead Sea salts

1 cup of coarse salts

½ cup of baking soda

1 cup of French green clay

5 drops of lavender essential oil

5 drops of clary sage essential oil

Moroccan Salt Soak

2 cups of Himalayan salts

1 cup of coarse sea salts

½ cup of baking soda

1 cup of rhassoul clay

handful of fresh rose petals

½ teaspoon of argan oil

10 drops of cedar essential oil

Himalayan Salt Soak

2 cups of Himalayan salts

1 cup of coarse sea salts

½ cup of baking soda

5 drops of jasmine essential oil

5 drops of spikenard essential oil

Hawaiian Salt Soak

2 cups of Himalayan salts

1 cup of coarse sea salts

½ cup of baking soda

10 drops of sandalwood essential oil

1 teaspoon of gardenia oil

1 teaspoon of kukui nut oil

African Salt Soak

2 cups of Dead Sea salts

1 cup of Epsom salts

½ cup of baking soda

5 drops of tea tree essential oil

5 drops of benzoin essential oil

1 teaspoon of baobab oil

CONCLUSION

My hope with this book is that you use it as your go-to guide when you need a little pick-me-up. We all have those days, don't we? Some of my most cherished books are the ones I've had for years that I always come back to when the need calls. So if you have a little ache or pain, or just need to de-stress, hopefully this will be your own cherished well-worn guide for years to come.

I've learned so much while doing research for this book, even beyond the properties of salts, oils, and scents. The most interesting aspect I've found is the effect these things have on our minds, which I'm finding more and more is the secret to good health! That's why baths are so powerful and healing. They not only nurture the body directly, but put your mind at ease, allowing it to regenerate.

While writing this book, an author who I've found extremely helpful in learning about the amazing healing capacities of essential oils is Patricia Davis. I have to thank her for the immense amount of information she provides in her books. If you are interested in learning more on how to use essential oils for healing and spiritual awareness, I highly Davis's *Aromatherapy: An A-Z*, *Subtle Aromatherapy*, and *Astrological Aromatherapy*.

Lastly, I truly believe this life is meant to be enjoyed. So most importantly, take time for yourself and be kind to your body.

CONVERSIONS

Common Conversions

1 gallon = 4 quarts = 8 pints = 16 cups = 128 fluid ounces = 3.8 liters
1 quart = 2 pints = 4 cups = 32 ounces = .95 liter
1 pint = 2 cups = 16 ounces = 480 ml
1 cup = 8 ounces = 240 ml
¼ cup = 4 tablespoons = 12 teaspoons = 2 ounces = 60 ml
1 tablespoon = 3 teaspoons = ½ fluid ounce = 15 ml

Volume Conversions

U.S.	U.S. EQUIVALENT	METRIC
1 tablespoon (3 teaspoons)	½ fluid ounce	15 milliliters
¼ cup	2 fluid ounces	60 milliliters
⅓ cup	3 fluid ounces	90 milliliters
½ cup	4 fluid ounces	120 milliliters
⅔ cup	5 fluid ounces	150 milliliters
¾ cup	6 fluid ounces	180 milliliters
1 cup	8 fluid ounces	240 milliliters
2 cups	16 fluid ounces	480 milliliters

INDEX

Aches and pains, and salt soaks, 47–48. *See also specific pains*
Acne: and bath bombs, 66; and salt scrubs, 65; and salt soaks, 65
Adrenal fatigue, 14
Ailment-related baths, 26–63; allergies, 27–28, 144; asthma, 28–29; athlete's foot, 29–30; chickenpox, 61–62; cystic fibrosis, 38–39; depression/fatigue, 56–58; fever, 42–43; headaches, 43–44; heart problems, 45-46; infections, 58–61, 63; inflammation, 46–47; pain, 47–53; respiratory issues, 30–37; skin problems, 54–55; stress, 39–41. *See also specific health concerns*
Allergies, and salt soaks, 27–28, 31, 144
Almond oil, 18
Antiaging baths: bath bombs, 67; salt scrubs, 67; salt soaks, 66–67

Aphrodisiac baths: bath bombs, 118; salt soaks, 125–29
Aquarius sun sign, 122–23
Aries sun sign, 107–108
Aromatherapy: An A-Z, 26, 167
"Around the world" soaks, 163–66
Arthritis, and salt soaks, 50–51
Asthma, and salt soaks, 28–29
Astrological Aromatherapy, 167
Astrology-related baths, 106–24; Aquarius, 122–23; Aries, 107–108; Cancer, 111–12; Capricorn, 120–21; Gemini, 110–11; Leo, 113–14; Libra, 116–17; Pisces, 123–24; Sagittarius, 119–20; Scorpio, 117–18; Taurus, 108–109; Virgo, 114–15
Athlete's foot, and salt soaks, 29–30
Aura chakra, 104–105
Avocado oil, 18

Back problems, and salt soaks, 49
Baking soda, 20

Index 171

Balance, importance, 12
Balancing baths: bath bombs, 69, 108, 121; salt scrubs, 68, 110; salt soaks, 68, 116
Base chakra, 94–95
Bath bombs: ingredients, 20; preparation and storage, 24. See also Bath treatments; see also specific bath bombs in Recipe Index
Bath salts: benefits, 12–14; types, 15
Bath treatments: ailments, 26–63; aphrodisiacs, 125–29; "around the world," 163–66; astrology, 106–24; benefits, 13–14; chakras, 93–105; floral, 154–62; ingredients, 15, 16–17, 18–20; meditative, 81–92; for men, 133–39; pregnancy, 130–34; preparation, 21–25; seasonal, 140–53; skin and beauty, 64–80
Beauty baths. See Skin and beauty baths; see also specific beauty concerns
Bergamot scent, 129
Blood pressure, and salt soaks, 45
Boils, and salt soaks, 54
Breathing problems. See Congestion; Respiratory issues
Bronchitis, and salt soaks, 32
Brow chakra, 101–102

Calming baths: bath bombs, 120, 162; salt scrubs, 158, 159; salt soaks, 40–41, 110, 157
Cancer sun sign, 111–12

Capricorn sun sign, 120–21
Carrier oils, 18–19
Cellulite: and bath bombs, 70; and salt scrubs, 69; and salt soaks, 69
Centering baths: salt soaks, 123
The Chakra Bible, 93
Chakra-related baths, 93–105; aura, 104–105; base, 94–95; brow, 101–102; crown, 103–104; heart, 98–99; sacral, 95–96; solar plexus, 97–98; throat, 100–101
Chakras for Beginners, 93
Chest congestion, and salt soaks, 29, 33, 39
Chickenpox, and salt soaks, 61–62
Citric acid, 20
Clays, 19–20
Cleansing baths: bath bombs, 71; salt scrubs, 71; salt soaks, 70, 108
Coconut oil, 19
Colds, and salt soaks: congestion, 33; disinfectant, 31; mucus, 35; prevention, 36–37
Comforting baths: salt scrubs, 91, 112; salt soaks, 88
Common colds. See Colds
Congestion, and salt soaks: allergies, 31; chest, 29, 33, 39; colds, 33; mucus 35
Cooling baths: bath bombs, 148; salt scrubs, 113; salt soaks, 147
Cough. See Dry cough; see also Congestion; Respiratory issues
Cracked skin. See Dry skin

Cramping, menstrual, and salt soaks, 52
Crown chakra, 103–104
Cystic fibrosis, and salt soaks, 38–39

Davis, Patricia, 12, 26, 93, 167
De-stressing. *See* Stress
Dead Sea salts, 15
Deep relaxation: salt scrubs, 91; salt soaks, 83, 117
Dehydrated skin. *See* Dry skin
Depression, and salt soaks, 56. *See also* Rejuvenating baths; Uplifting baths
Detoxifying baths: bath bombs, 72; salt scrubs, 72; salt soaks, 50, 71
Dry cough, and salt soaks, 32, 35
Dry skin: and bath bombs, 74, 76; and salt scrubs, 74, 76; and salt soaks, 72–74, 75. *See also* Eczema

Eczema: and bath bombs, 75; and salt soaks, 74–75
Epsom salts, 15
Equipment, for preparation, 22, 23, 24
Essential oils, 26; benefits, 16–17; precautions, 17, 130

Fall baths, 150–53
Fatigue, mental, and salt scrubs, 58; and salt soaks, 57
Fatigue, physical, and salt soaks, 49, 56
Fever, and salt soaks, 42–43

Fight-or-flight mode, 13–14
Floral baths, 154–62; bath bombs, 159–62; salt scrubs, 157–59; salt soaks, 154–57
Floral powders, 24
Flu, and salt soaks: congestion, 33; disinfectant, 31; infection, 34; prevention, 36–37, 141
Food coloring, 24
French green clay, 19
Fuller's earth clay, 20

Gemini sun sign, 110–11
Grounding baths: bath bombs, 90, 112; salt scrubs, 122; salt soaks, 85

Hay fever. *See* Allergies
Headaches, and salt soaks, 43–44
Heart chakra, 98–99
Heart problems, and salt soaks, 45–46
Hemorrhoids, and salt soaks, 62
Himalayan salts, 15

Immune system, and salt soaks, 60
Infections, and salt soaks, 58–61, 63. *See also* Respiratory infections
Inflammation, and salt soaks, 46–47
Influenza. *See* Flu
Ingredients, of baths, 15, 16–17, 18–20
Intentions, setting, 12, 81–82; and chakras, 93
Intoxicating baths: salt scrubs, 118

Index 173

Invigorating baths: bath bombs, 88; salt scrubs, 92, 119
Itching, and salt scrubs/soaks, 55

Jars, for storage, 22
Jasmine scent, 127
Jojoba oil, 19

Kukui nut oil, 19

Leo sun sign, 113–14
Libra sun sign, 116–17
Lymphatic system, and salt soaks, 59

Meditation, 81
Meditative baths, 81–92; bath bombs, 88–90; salt scrubs, 91–92; and salt soaks, 83–88, 122
Men, and baths, 133–39
Menstrual cramping, and salt soaks, 52
Mental fatigue: and salt scrubs, 58; salt soaks, 57
Mercier, Patricia, 93
Minerals, 13
Moisturizing baths: bath bombs, 76; salt scrubs, 76; salt soaks, 75
Moods. *See* Rejuvenating baths; Uplifting baths
Mountain Rose Herbs (company), 17
Mucus, expelling, and salt soak, 35
Muscles, and salt soaks, 48

Nurturing baths: salt soaks, 114

Oily skin: and bath bombs, 78; and salt scrubs, 78; and salt soaks, 77
Olive oil, 19

Pain, and salt soaks, 47–53. *See also specific pains* (Aches; Cramping; etc.)
Painful periods, and salt soaks, 52
Pampering baths: salt soaks, 120
Patchouli scent, 128
Pisces sun sign, 123–24
PMS, and salt soaks, 52–53
Pond, David, 93
Pregnancy: and baths, 130–34; and essential oils, 17, 130
Preparation, of baths, 21–25

Re-balancing baths. *See* Balancing baths
Rejuvenating baths: bath bombs, 147; salt scrubs, 57, 146; salt soaks, 57, 146
Relaxing baths: bath bombs, 111; salt scrubs, 91, 158; salt soaks, 83, 117
Repetitive strain, and salt soaks, 48
Replenishing baths: salt soaks, 119
Respiratory issues, and salt soaks, 30–37
Restoring baths: salt scrubs, 158
Reviving baths: salt scrubs, 121
Rhassoul clay, 20
Rose scent, 126
Rosehip oil, 19

Sacral chakra, 95–96

Sagittarius sun sign, 119–20
Salt scrubs: ingredients, 18–19; preparation and storage, 23–24. See also Bath treatments; see also specific salt scrubs in Recipe Index
Salt soaks: ingredients, 15, 19–20; preparation and storage, 21–23. See also Bath treatments; see also specific salt soaks in Recipe Index
Salts, bath: benefits, 12–14; types, 15
Sciatica, and salt soaks, 49
Scorpio sun sign, 117–18
Sea salts. See Salts, bath
Seasonal baths, 140–53; fall, 150–53; spring, 144–47; summer, 147–50; winter, 140–43
Sensitive skin: and bath bombs, 79; and salt soaks, 79
Sesame oil, 19
Skin and beauty baths, 64–80; acne, 65–66; antiaging, 66–67; cellulite, 69–70; cleansing, 70–72; dry skin, 72–76; oily skin, 77–78; sensitive skin, 79; skin-balancing, 68–69. See also specific skin concerns
Skin-balancing baths: bath bombs, 69; salt scrubs, 68; salt soaks, 68
Skin smoothing baths: bath bombs, 80; salt scrubs, 80; salt soaks, 79
Solar plexus chakra, 97–98
Soothing baths: salt scrubs, 107; salt soaks, 107

Spasms, and salt soaks, 28, 49, 50
Spring baths, 144–47
Storage, 22, 23, 24; jars, 22
Stimulating baths: bath bombs, 109
Stress, 13–14; and bath bombs, 40; and salt scrubs, 40; and salt soaks, 39, 40
Subtle Aromatherapy, 12, 93, 167
Summer baths, 147–50
Sun signs, and baths, 106–24. See also specific signs
Sunburn, and salt soaks, 54
Sunflower oil, 19

Tachycardia, and salt soaks, 45–46
Taurus sun sign, 108–109
Tendinitis, and salt soaks, 47
Throat chakra, 100–101
Tiredness. See Fatigue

Uplifting baths: bath bombs, 114, 123, 143; salt scrubs, 56, 92, 143; salt soaks, 84, 113
Urinary tract infections, and salt soaks, 59–60

Varicose veins, and salt soaks, 63
Viral infection, and salt soaks, 61
Virgo sun sign, 114–15

Warming baths: bath bombs, 113, 142; salt scrubs, 142; salt soaks, 142
Winter baths, 140–43

Yeast infections, and salt soaks, 63

RECIPE INDEX

Acne Bath Bomb, 66
Acne Purifying Salt Soaks, 65
Acne Salt Scrub, 65
African Salt Soak, 166
Allergy Salt Soaks, 27–28
Ancient Egyptian Salt Soak, 164
Ancient Roman Salt Soak, 164
Antiaging Bath Bomb, 67
Antiaging Salt Scrub, 67
Antiaging Salt Soaks, 66–67
Antibacterial Salt Soaks, 58
Antidepressant Salt Soak, 56
Anti-Inflammation Salt Soak, 46
Aquarius Grounding Salt Scrub, 122
Aquarius Meditating Salt Soak, 122
Aquarius Uplifting Bath Bomb, 123
Aries Balancing Bath Bomb, 108
Aries Restoring Salt Scrub, 107
Aries Soothing Salt Soak, 107
Arthritis Salt Soak for Circulation, 50
Asthma Salt Soaks, 28–29
Athlete's Foot Salt Soaks, 29–30

Aura Chakra Bath Bomb, 105
Aura Chakra Salt Scrub, 104
Aura Chakra Salt Soak, 104

Backache Salt Soaks…, 49
Base Chakra Bath Bomb, 95
Base Chakra Salt Scrub, 94
Base Chakra Salt Soak, 94
Beach Bath Bomb, 150
Beach Salt Scrub, 149
Beach Salt Soak, 149
Bedtime Bath Bomb, 89
Bergamot and Jasmine Salt Soak, 87
Bergamot Grounding Salt Soak, 85
Bergamot Salt Scrub, 138
Bergamot Salt Soak, 129
Brighter Days Bath Bomb, 145
Brighter Days Salt Scrub, 144
Brighter Days Salt Soak, 144
Bronchitis Salt Soaks for Dry Cough, 32
Brow Chakra Bath Bomb, 102
Brow Chakra Salt Scrub, 102

Brow Chakra Salt Soak, 101

Calendula Bath Bomb, 161
Calendula Salt Soak, 156
Calming Floral Bath Bomb, 162
Calming Floral Blend, 157
Calming Floral Salt Scrub, 159
Calming Salt Soaks, 40–41
Cancer Comforting Salt Scrub, 112
Cancer Grounding Bath Bomb, 112
Cancer Serene Salt Soak, 111
Capricorn Balancing Bath Bomb, 121
Capricorn Pampering Salt Soak, 120
Capricorn Reviving Salt Scrub, 121
Cedarwood and Bergamot Salt Soak, 136
Cedarwood and Lavender Salt Soak, 87
Cedarwood Bath Bomb, 139
Cellulite Bath Bomb, 70
Cellulite Salt Scrub, 69
Cellulite Salt Soak, 69
Chamomile Bath Bomb, 160
Chamomile Salt Soak, 155
Chickenpox Salt Soaks, 61–62
Citronella Uplifting Salt Soak, 84
Clary Sage and Lavender Salt Soak, 136
Clary Sage Salt Scrub, 138
Clary Sage Uplifting Salt Soak, 84
Cleansing Bath Bomb, 71
Cleansing Salt Scrub, 71
Cleansing Salt Soak, 70
Cold and Flu Congestion Salt Soaks, 33
Comforting Benzoin Salt Soak, 88

Comforting Salt Scrub, 91
Common Cold Salt Soaks, 36–37
Congestion Salt Soak, 31
Cooling Summer Bath Bomb, 148
Cooling Summer Salt Soak, 147
Cracked-Skin Salt Soaks, 72–73
Crown Chakra Bath Bomb, 104
Crown Chakra Salt Scrub, 103
Crown Chakra Salt Soak, 103
Cystic Fibrosis Salt Soaks, 38–39

Deep Relaxation Salt Scrub, 91
Dehydrated-Skin Salt Soak, 73
Delicate Floral Bath Bomb, 162
Delicate Floral Blend Salt Soak, 156
Delicate Floral Salt Scrub, 157
Delicate Jasmine Salt Soak, 127
De-stress Bath Bomb, 40
De-stress Salt Scrub, 40
De-stress Salt Soaks, 39
Detoxifying Arthritis Salt Soak, 50
Detoxifying Bath Bomb, 72
Detoxifying Salt Scrub, 72
Detoxifying Salt Soak, 71
Disinfectant Salt Soak…, 31
Dry-Skin Bath Bomb, 74
Dry-Skin Salt Scrub, 74
Dry-Skin Salt Soak, 73
Dull Aches and Pains Salt Soak, 47

Eczema Bath Bomb, 75
Eczema Salt Soaks, 74–75
Exotic Spring Bath Bomb, 146
Exotic Spring Salt Scrub, 145
Exotic Spring Salt Soak, 145

Fall Comfort Bath Bomb, 151

Fall Comfort Salt Scrub, 151
Fall Comfort Salt Soak, 150
Fatigue Salt Soak, 56
Fever-Reducing Salt Soaks, 42–43
Frankincense and Benzoin Salt Soak, 137
French Salt Soak, 165

Gemini Balancing Salt Scrub, 110
Gemini Calming Salt Soak, 110
Gemini Relaxing Bath Bomb, 111
Gentle Calendula Salt Scrub, 158
Gentle Salt Scrub, 92
Geranium and Chamomile Salt Soak, 86
Grapefruit and Rose Bath Bomb, 89
Grounding Bath Bomb, 90

Hawaiian Salt Soak, 166
Headache Salt Soaks, 43–44
Heart Chakra Bath Bomb, 99
Heart Chakra Salt Scrub, 99
Heart Chakra Salt Soak, 98
Hemorrhoids Salt Soaks, 62
High Blood Pressure Salt Soak, 45
Himalayan Salt Soak, 165

Immunity Salt Soaks, 60
Influenza Salt Soaks, 34
Invigorating Bath Bomb, 88
Invigorating Salt Scrub, 92

Jasmine Bath Bomb, 159
Jasmine Salt Soak, 156

Lavender Bath Bomb, 161

Lavender Pregnancy Bath Bomb, 134
Lavender Pregnancy Salt Scrub, 133
Lavender Pregnancy Salt Soak, 133
Lavender Relaxation Salt Scrub, 158
Lavender Salt Soak, 155
Leo Cooling Salt Scrub, 113
Leo Uplifting Bath Bomb, 114
Leo Warming Salt Soak, 113
Libra Beautifying Salt Scrub, 116
Libra Luxurious Bath Bomb, 117
Libra Rebalancing Salt Soak, 116
Low Blood Pressure Salt Soak, 45
Lymphatic Cleanse Salt Soak, 59

Mental Fatigue Salt Scrub, 58
Mental Fatigue Salt Soak, 57
Modern Roman Salt Soak, 164
Moisturizing Bath Bomb, 76
Moisturizing Salt Scrub, 76
Moisturizing Salt Soak, 75
Moroccan Salt Soak, 165
Muscle Pain Salt Soak, 48
Muscle Relaxer Salt Soak, 48

Neroli and Mandarin Pregnancy Bath Bomb, 131
Neroli and Mandarin Pregnancy Salt Scrub, 131
Neroli and Mandarin Pregnancy Salt Soak, 131

Oily Skin Bath Bomb, 78
Oily Skin Salt Scrubs, 78
Oily Skin Salt Soaks, 77

Painful Periods Salt Soaks, 52

Pain-Reducing Arthritis Salt Soaks, 51
Patchouli and Oakmoss Salt Soak, 137
Patchouli Deep Relaxation Salt Soak, 83
Patchouli Salt Soak, 128
Peppermint Bath Bomb, 139
Pisces Centering Salt Soak, 123
Pisces Dreamy Bath Bomb, 124
Pisces Therapeutic Salt Scrub, 124
PMS Salt Soaks, 52–53

Rejuvenating Salt Scrub, 57
Rejuvenating Salt Soak, 57
Rejuvenating Spring Bath Bomb, 147
Rejuvenating Spring Salt Scrub, 146
Rejuvenating Spring Salt Soak, 146
Repetitive Strain Injury Salt Soak, 48
Respiratory Salt Soaks, 30–31
Rose and Basil Salt Soak, 85
Rose and Chamomile Pregnancy Bath Bomb, 133
Rose and Chamomile Pregnancy Salt Scrub, 132
Rose and Chamomile Pregnancy Salt Soak, 132
Rose Bath Bomb, 160
Rose Restoring Salt Scrub, 158
Rose Salt Soak, 126, 155
Rosemary Bath Bomb, 138

Sacral Chakra Bath Bomb, 96
Sacral Chakra Salt Scrub, 96
Sacral Chakra Salt Soak, 95
Sagittarius Calming Bath Bomb, 120

Sagittarius Invigorating Salt Scrub, 119
Sagittarius Replenishing Salt Soak, 119
Salt Soak for Boils, 54
Salt Soaks for Expelling Mucus, 35
Sciatica Salt Soak, 49
Scorpio Aphrodisiac Bath Bomb, 118
Scorpio Deep Relaxation Salt Soak, 117
Scorpio Intoxicating Salt Scrub, 118
Sensitive Skin Bath Bomb, 79
Sensitive Skin Salt Soak, 79
Sharp Aches and Pains Salt Soak, 47
Simple Calming Chamomile Salt Scrub, 158
Skin-Balancing Bath Bomb, 69
Skin-Balancing Salt Scrub, 68
Skin-Balancing Salt Soak, 68
Skin-Smoothing Bath Bomb, 80
Skin-Smoothing Salt Scrub, 80
Skin-Smoothing Salt Soak, 80
Solar Plexus Chakra Bath Bomb, 98
Solar Plexus Chakra Salt Scrub, 97
Solar Plexus Chakra Salt Soak, 97
Soothing Frankincense Salt Soak, 86
Soothing Salt Scrubs for Itching, 55
Soothing Salt Soak for Itching, 55
Spicy Fall Bath Bomb, 153
Spicy Fall Salt Scrub, 153
Spicy Fall Salt Soak, 152
Stimulating Bath Bomb, 90
Summer Holiday Bath Bomb, 149
Summer Holiday Salt Scrub, 148
Summer Holiday Salt Soak, 148
Sunburn Salt Soak, 54

Tachycardia Salt Soaks, 45–46
Taurus Cleansing Salt Soak, 108
Taurus Luxurious Salt Scrub, 109
Taurus Stimulating Bath Bomb, 109
Tea Tree Salt Scrub, 137
Tendinitis Salt Soak, 47
Throat Chakra Bath Bomb, 101
Throat Chakra Salt Scrub, 100
Throat Chakra Salt Soak, 100

Uplifting Mood Salt Scrub, 56
Uplifting Salt Scrub, 92
Uplifting Winter Bath Bomb, 143
Uplifting Winter Salt Scrub, 143
Uplifting Winter Salt Soak, 143
Urinary Tract Infection Salt Soaks, 59–60

Varicose Veins Salt Soak, 63
Viral Infection Salt Soaks, 61
Virgo Healing Bath Bomb, 115
Virgo Indulgence Salt Scrub, 115
Virgo Nurturing Salt Soak, 114

Warming Winter Bath Bomb, 142
Warming Winter Salt Scrub, 142
Warming Winter Salt Soak, 142
Winter Flu Prevention Bath Bomb, 141
Winter Flu Prevention Salt Soak, 141
Woodsy Fall Bath Bomb, 152
Woodsy Fall Salt Scrub, 152
Woodsy Fall Salt Soak, 151

Yeast Infection Salt Soak, 63

ACKNOWLEDGMENTS

For my parents, who raised me to be independent and go for my dreams rather than play it safe. Thanks for your support and guidance—it seems to be working.

ABOUT THE AUTHOR

Kate Bello is a writer and photographer living in San Diego, California. With a background in media design and an interest in wellness, Kate started blogging in 2008 about homemade beauty and healthy recipes. Since then she has written for *Thoughtfully Magazine, Somerset Home, Willow and Sage,* and *Artful Blogging* and received Editor's Favorite for her photography on National Geographic's Your Shot.